# Occupational Therapy and Spirituality

Spirituality is an important aspect of occupational therapy theory and practice, yet it remains little understood.

This timely book adds to the current debate by exploring the meaning of spirituality within occupational therapy and by outlining evidence which supports this area of practice. Beginning with the three stances surrounding spirituality for the common good and the theology of occupation, throughout its 10 chapters the book goes on to cover topics such as:

- Spirituality of caring;
- Theories of spiritual development;
- Definition of spirituality from occupational therapy literature;
- Differences between assessing spirituality and religion;
- Spirituality and ethics;
- Spiritual and cultural diversity in the occupational therapy clinic;
- Therapeutic self.

By the end of the volume the reader will have the toolset required to consider spiritual concepts and their application to health principles. *Occupational Therapy and Spirituality* is written in an accessible format and is designed for occupational therapy and occupational science academics, researchers, and graduate students.

**Barbara Hemphill** is Associate Professor Emeritus at Western Michigan University. Dr. Hemphill was appointed to the State of Michigan Ethics Board for Occupational Therapists and was elected Chair of the Ethics Commission to the American Occupational Therapy Association in 2009.

# Routledge Advances in Occupational Science and Occupational Therapy

**Occupational Therapy and Spirituality**
*Barbara Hemphill*

For more information about this series, please visit: www.routledge.com/ Routledge-Advances-in-Occupational-Science-and-Occupational-Therapy/book-series/RAOSOT

# Occupational Therapy and Spirituality

Barbara Hemphill

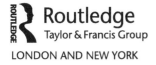

Routledge
Taylor & Francis Group

LONDON AND NEW YORK

First published 2020
by Routledge
4 Park Square, Milton Park, Abingdon, Oxon OX14 4RN
605 Third Avenue, New York, NY 10017

First issued in paperback 2023

*Routledge is an imprint of the Taylor & Francis Group, an informa business*

*British Library Cataloguing-in-Publication Data*
A catalogue record for this book is available from the British Library

*Library of Congress Cataloging-in-Publication Data*
A catalog record for this book has been requested

ISBN: 978-1-03-257076-1 (pbk)
ISBN: 978-0-367-22807-1 (hbk)
ISBN: 978-0-429-27693-4 (ebk)

DOI: 10.4324/9780429276934

Typeset in Times New Roman
by Wearset Ltd, Boldon, Tyne and Wear

Publisher's Note
The publisher has gone to great lengths to ensure the quality of this reprint but
points out that some imperfections in the original copies may be apparent.

# Contents

# A message to the reader

I have a body, but I am not my body; I am more than that.

My body may be in different conditions of health or sickness.

It may be rested or tired, but it is not my real "I."

My body is my precious instrument of experience and of action, but I am not my body.

I am more than that. I am the one who is aware.

I have emotions, but I am more than my emotions.

They are countless, contradictory, changing,

And yet I know that I always remain I, my self, in a state of irritation or calm.

Since I can observe, understand, and judge my emotions and then increasingly dominate, direct, and utilize them, it is evident that they are not my self.

I have emotions, but I am not my emotion. I am more than that; I am the one who is aware.

I have intellect, but I am more than my intellect. It may be quiet or active.

It is capable of expanding, letting go of limiting beliefs, and learning new attitudes.

It is an organ of knowledge in regard to the inner world as well as the outer.

But it is not my self.

I have an intellect, but I am not my intellect. I am more than that. I am the one who is aware.

I am the center of pure self-awareness. I am the center of will.

Capable of mastering and directing all my energies:

Physical, emotional, mental, and spiritual.

I am the one who is aware. I am the self.

(Adapted from R. Assagioli (1973), *The Act of Will*, New York: Penguin, pp. 214–217)

# Foreword

Barbara J. Hemphill is highly qualified to be the author of this work. A long career as an occupational therapist and educator led her to develop and address her own spiritual journey. After retiring as a full-time university faculty member, she continued a full professional life, in part by pursuing graduate study in clerical ministry. In 2004 she earned a doctoral degree in ministry from the Ecumenical Theology Seminary in Detroit. Her dissertation was concerned with the spiritual development of occupational therapy students. She has had a long and stellar career as a writer of published works in occupational therapy, particularly works devoted to assessments used in mental health. No one is more qualified to address the area of spirituality.

In a quest for a full understanding of occupation and how it translates into therapy, occupational therapists have thought, discussed, and written extensively about their therapeutic domain. The domain (American Occupational Therapy Association, 2008), and its first edition, include spirituality as an important portion of life and health to be considered and addressed. There are some, but not many, publications that deal with spirituality as a practical matter in therapeutic situations. We now have a thoughtful and thorough approach to this gap.

After laying groundwork on the meaning and role of occupation itself, Professor Hemphill carefully differentiates between spirituality and religion. The book addresses various aspects of religious beliefs and practices, though it sees spirituality as a larger issue, one which explains and engages the core concerns of many non-believers.

Crucial attention is given to how spirituality relates to the therapeutic use of self and the relationship of this concept to caring. The book incorporates many concepts from writings of occupational therapists about spirituality, bringing them together with her fresh approach to the topic.

Hemphill also discusses varying faith traditions, describing many of the practices of important religious cohorts in the United States and elsewhere. There is a thorough discussion of ethics in occupational therapy and their relationship to morality and spirituality. Here again, the author is eminently qualified to address issues of ethics. Of particular value is the careful delineation of steps to be taken when the therapist (or anyone else, for that matter) faces an ethical dilemma. This is the most complete set of ideas encountered to this point of going about the assessment of and then acting on an ethical dilemma. This is only a partial description of the many important ideas included in Hemphill's comprehensive work.

Among its accomplishments is the fact that the book deals with both physical and mental health and how the provision of occupational therapy relates to questions raised in the totality of intervention. Concepts are clearly defined throughout. The book also presents assessments that can be used to determine areas of spirituality that could affect intervention. And an additional major accomplishment is its presentation of approaches to teaching occupational therapists and others about how spirituality relates to practice. It includes a discussion of classroom expectations and the presentation of relevant concepts to students.

This book is a memorable contribution to occupational therapy literature. It is written in a clear and straightforward manner and its content is highly practical. It should stimulate discussion of many aspects of spirituality and its role in occupational therapy.

Marie-Louise Blount
Co-Editor, *Occupational Therapy in Mental Health*

## Reference

American Occupational Therapy Association (2008). Occupational therapy practice framework: Domain and process (2nd ed.). *American Journal of Occupational Therapy, 62*, 625–683.

# Preface

We are spirits having a human experience.

(Anonymous)

## Faith journey

For most of my professional life, I have taught occupational therapy students and practiced in mental health. I am on a spiritual journey that involves a reciprocal relationship between my professional life and my religious life. In tandem with my professional career growth, spiritual experiences affected my worldview. That reciprocal relationship created in me an awareness of the spiritual dimension in the practice of occupational therapy, a profession that recognizes the whole person.

Since my retirement, I have continued on that spiritual journey, which now manifests itself through my pursuit of an understanding of spirituality in the clinical environment and in educating occupational therapy students. Everyone is born of spirit, and patients who seek medical assistance and students who are admitted to occupational therapy programs are at various levels of spiritual development.

I was born and educated in the Midwest. My own faith journey began in the Evangelical United Brethren Church, where I was baptized and received my catechism (also known as a book, giving a brief summary of the basic principles of Christianity in question-and-answer form). My paternal grandfather provided my religious instruction and was the most influential person in my religious development. Like many youths, I left home after high school to pursue my life's work. I occasionally sought spiritual guidance, but in general I did not attend religious services regularly.

During the first half of my life, I focused my energies on establishing a career. In 1968, I received by Bachelor of Science (BS) in occupational therapy from the University of Iowa. I worked as an occupational therapist until 1976, when I received my Master's degree in occupational therapy from Colorado State University. My interest was in projective media—a technique that uses art to help patients express their thoughts and feelings. This resulted in a study that examined the reliability of an assessment called the BH Battery (Hemphill, 1982).

Early in my career, during my tenure as an occupational therapist at Fort Logan Mental Health Center, I was fortunate enough to work with Maxwell Jones, the founder of the therapeutic community concept in mental health (Jacobs & Jacobs, 2004). As a clinician, I supervised personnel and guided occupational therapy students in the mental health treatment of young adults and, especially, older adults. This experience helped me understand the significance of community and influenced my thinking about spiritual development.

In 1975, I began my teaching career at Cleveland State University in the occupational therapy program, where I stayed until 1981, when I became an associate professor in the Department of Occupational Therapy at Western Michigan University (WMU). At WMU, my primary responsibilities were conducting research and teaching occupational therapy theory and assessments in mental health to undergraduate and graduate students. I was tenured in 1985 and am presently retired with the rank of associate professor emeritus.

I married late in life, to a man who believed he was on a spiritual journey. This intrigued me and I was eager to learn more about this journey. Soon after our marriage, it became apparent to me that I needed to pursue my own spiritual journey before I could deal effectively with patients' spiritual needs and teach health care students how to do the same. Accordingly, I became more involved with my faith community. In this environment, I was able to pursue my spiritual needs independently without being judged by anyone that may not understand such a journey. My husband and I wanted to study spiritual concepts, so we selected attending a meeting that studied the Course in Miracles (a new-age spirituality). In addition to the Course in Miracles, I also studied the Bible.

The Course in Miracles helped me recognize my spiritual journey and my relationship with my Creator, my students, my professional life, and my overall worldview. I attended study groups and workshops as well as week-long retreats. At a workshop that had me struggling with many of the concepts presented, I experienced a "mountaintop" event: I believe that I encountered my Creator. I have not openly always shared this experience. It certainly made me a believer, and it has had a profound effect on my life and religious faith. This experience directly influenced my relationship with students as well as my attitude toward teaching. It made me realize the impact spirituality can have on patients and the importance of spiritual development for health care professionals.

## Teaching spirituality in the classroom

As a result of my mountaintop experience, I began to look at the course content I was teaching and to integrate spiritual concepts into my courses. In addition, I came to believe that for educators, the personal spiritual journey must include a commitment to students about embarking on their own spiritual journey. If health care professionals are to establish a relationship with their patients, it is important that they recognize how a spiritual journey affects their relationships with their Creator, family, and other people. I was always careful not to speak of religious doctrine. I used published occupational therapy literature and an audiotape of Bernie Siegel's (1990) *Love, Medicine and Miracles.* At the end of the semester, my students were required to address the question "What role does spirituality have in the practice of occupational therapy?" The feedback from students about the course was positive, and they seemed to understand how spirituality could affect patients' treatment. I felt I had successfully taught spirituality in the classroom without offending students' religious beliefs.

My 24 years as a faculty member have given me the opportunity to work with students and scholars in my professional field. I have accomplished much, and I hope to accomplish more in my retirement. In part because of my clinical experience and my work with the Course in Miracles, I believe that a spiritual dimension is essential in the clinical environment and the education of occupational therapy students. Therefore, during the years I spent teaching, I searched for a method of integrating spirituality into the classroom. In that search, I came to believe that spirituality manifests itself in a concept that was part of the profession's early development. That concept, coupled with the idea of appropriate treatment for patients is the *therapeutic use of self.* The self makes a critical difference in successful treatment, and the use of self operationalizes spirituality in the therapeutic process. The use of self and a meaningful occupation act as the vehicles through which the client expresses his or her spirituality. The therapeutic self is further discussed in this text. During my professional career I became interested in mental health assessments in which I edited a number of books. I was recognized for my contribution to education, research, and publication by receiving the Distinguished Roster of Fellows from the American Occupational Therapy Association and Distinguished Roster of Fellows of the Michigan Occupational Therapy Association.

## Spirituality in the clinic

While working with patients and students, I became convinced that theories and techniques of practice do not alone help a patient become successful at living a meaningful life. In my experience, some patients get better and others did not, even though techniques, theories, and principles of treatment were the same. It seemed to me that another factor influenced treatment. As a therapist, I was interested in projective media, through which patients can project their innermost thoughts and feelings. I found that patients expressed religious themes most often during assessment time, using finger-painting. When finger-painting was used as a meaningful occupation for expressing spirituality, it became important and allowed patients to express their innermost self. Early in my career, the field did not view religious themes in evaluation and treatment as legitimate concerns. I could interpret these themes from the literature, but I was unable to use my knowledge in treating patients until later in my career. These experiences and my own faith journey led me to pursue my interest in spirituality further in occupational therapy.

## Occupational therapy, spirituality, and holism

Embedded in the philosophy of occupational therapy is the concept of *holism*: that therapists attend to clients' mind, body, and spirit. As a teacher, I did not find it difficult to teach students about illness and disease from a physical and psychological perspective. As the years went by, however, it became clear that the spirit part of the triad is missing.

The mind–body–spirit triad is an important concept in occupational therapy. The phrase *treating the person holistically* describes a treatment process in which the therapist considers clients' physical, emotional, intellectual, social, spiritual, and lifestyle dimensions (Reed & Sanderson, 1999). Reed and Sanderson (1999) wrote that "the environment includes internal (body) and external (human and non-human) aspects" (p. 217). The concept of holism promotes clients' determination of their own state of health. The process of treatment—of achieving health—involves the interaction among systems of the body, the therapist, and the client's relationship to the world. Reed and Sanderson (1999) stated, "The belief that a person should be integrated as a whole is very consistent with the philosophy of an occupational therapist, which states that the therapist work with the whole person" (p. 218). Holism is not a new concept; it has ancient origins. In Chapter 3, I describe the theology of the body and soul and discuss its relationship to modern-day occupational therapy practice.

Holistic treatment includes the client's spirit as well as his or her body and mind, but the spiritual aspect of the holistic dimension has been neglected in the treatment process and in the education of occupational therapy students. I therefore began to integrate the spiritual dimension into my classroom and patient practice. As I progressed on my own spiritual journey, I began to confidently integrate the use of projective media as a method of accessing the patient's spiritual self.

The official documents throughout the history of occupational therapy promote a holistic perspective as the hallmark of the profession. The field, however, has no official definition of spirituality related to the practice of occupational therapy. Although spirituality is included in the *Occupational Therapy Practice Framework* (American Occupational Therapy Association [AOTA], 2008, 2014), the *Framework* does not present a workable and definitive process for using spirituality in practice. As a result, I began to review the religious and professional literature. In an attempt to define spirituality in the context of occupational therapy, this book presents spirituality and its development from the perspective of various religious traditions, as reflected in social and medical professional, lay, and occupational therapy literature.

## Spiritual development

Understanding one's own spiritual development can be seen as an important part of being a therapist. Mosey (1986) stated that "the conscious use of self involves planning one's personal responses so as to help a patient" (p. 42). Everyone is on a spiritual journey at some level—be it conscious or unconscious—and that spiritual journey is expressed through everyday activities and the person's religious tradition. Therefore, when students come to the occupational therapy program or therapists come to the clinic, they are at some level of spiritual development. Through study and awareness, the student or therapist may become aware of his or her own spiritual development and its impact on the client during the therapeutic process. It is important that the therapist in training develops and becomes aware of his or her own spiritual path. I believe that awareness of a spiritual path helps therapists integrate spirituality into the treatment process, which may enhance the client's outcome. Consequently, I believe that teaching spirituality in the classroom is an important aspect of occupational therapy education. This book therefore reviews the prominent development theories of spirituality, as articulated by Fowler (1981), Moody and Carroll (1997), and Peck (1987, 1997).

My concern is not for people who come to occupational therapy with a solid religious tradition but for those who state, "I'm spiritual but not religious." It is important, in my judgment, that both students and therapists be able to recognize their stage of spiritual development and their spiritual journey and to take an interfaith approach to client treatment. Understanding one's own spiritual development is a major theme of this book.

## Spirit as an occupation

*Occupational therapy* is a health profession that promotes the use of occupation to assist people throughout the lifespan with adapting to the environment for the purpose of achieving quality of life. Occupation is the science, and occupational therapy is the profession that applies the science of occupation. *Occupational science* is a social and behavioral science that studies individuals as doers with disabilities and how they adapt to situations in the environment through occupations. That is, they can adapt through deliberate, mindful, organized action. The field of occupational therapy emphasized adapting while engaging in an activity; this results in quality of life (Zemke & Clark, 1996). What is quality of life to one person may be different to another. Christiansen and Baum (1997) stated that quality of life is defined by the patient's perception of performance in four areas: (1) physical and occupational function, (2) psychological state of mind, (3) social interaction, and (4) somatic and bodily state. Spirituality can be included in any one of these four areas.

Occupations are expressed symbolically in a culture and are interpreted in the context of people's life stories. Wilcock (1989) proposed a theory of occupation that examines human nature from a biological and social perspective. Wilcock (2006) stated that occupational imbalances, occupational deprivation, and occupational alienation are best addressed by creating an environment in which people "experience satisfaction, purpose, meaning, and ongoing health and well-being through what they do" (p. 11). To have *occupational balance* means to have a state of emotional and mental stability, and be able to make rational decisions and judgments. It is a balance between intrinsic and extrinsic factors.

*Occupational deprivation* means to be deprived of the ability to acquire, use, or enjoy something—for example, one's need to worship or establish a relationship with a transcendent being. *Occupational alienation* is a phenomenon whereby humans are estranged from following their human nature. People can be alienated from the activity of their economic, social, and spiritual nature (Wilcock, 2006). Spirit, viewed as an occupation, may pursue an equilibrium between mental and emotional state, may pursue enjoyment with the transcendent being, and achieve the ability to pursue human fulfillment.

Quality of life can be defined as "a state of well-being and functioning that includes a level of comfort, enjoyment, and ability to participate in meaningful activities or occupations" (Crepeau, Cohn, & Schell, 2003, p. 1033). To achieve quality of life, spirituality may be viewed as an essential aspect of the quality of life triadic. There is no hierarchy. Spiritual quality of life is achieved through interconnectedness among humans, the world, and a transcendent being—or among the client, the therapist, and a higher power.

Spirituality is experienced in the context of the inner self and the outer world and is expressed through action in the world. Health care services are carried out in the context of the treatment setting and are consciously and unconsciously influenced by the client's beliefs, perceptions, and culture. The client's culture and customs are grounded in the external world and influence how services are delivered. The process of knowing the client's inner world and how that world is expressed in the outer world is a concept I call the *theology of occupation*; I devote an entire chapter to presenting this concept.

## Therapeutic ministry

In my journey, I have grown to believe that the therapeutic self is a type of ministry that manifests itself in the relationship established between therapist and client during the therapeutic process. I am a dedicated professional who also wants to give my students the tools that will help them become effective therapists. Therefore, I integrated the concept of spirituality, through the concept of the therapeutic use of self, into my courses using projective media, in the hope that my students would learn that the interaction between client and therapist is an important element in successful practice.

Throughout my teaching career, however, I have had to be careful about what I taught in regard to the content of spirituality. Even though WMU includes a Department of Comparative Religion, its faculty was hesitant about teaching religious concepts and felt to do so would be in conflict with the Department of Holistic Health. Working in a state- and federally supported institution, I had to teach about spirituality without espousing a particular religious doctrine. Engel (1974) spelled out guidelines for teaching spirituality, and I followed them. In addition, I found it important to distinguish between spirituality and holistic health. Holistic health is a discipline in itself. The spiritual concept in holistic health is too broad and too generic to be helpful in the occupational therapy treatment process. Many of the interventions used in holistic health, such as acupuncture and meditation, are not a part of occupational therapy's legitimate toolbox. Spirituality in the context of occupational therapy is more specific and includes broad religious concepts that will be explained in this book.

As a retired person who continues to be deeply committed to the profession, my interest in spirituality manifests in the therapeutic use of self-concept. My interest in spirituality has developed, grown, and deepened for me, personally. I am a clinician who wants to be effective with clients and an educator who wants students to learn. To be successful, the therapist–educator must integrate religious theology with treatment principles that manifest in the therapeutic self. This interest has led me to believe that the occupational therapy field needed to examine the value of spirituality in the education of its students and that doing so would enhance success in treatment. It is important to know whether students and therapists are really learning to use themselves therapeutically. Because I am no longer involved on a daily basis in occupational therapy education, I believe I may have a deeper perspective on the profession as well as the luxury of being able to take a step back.

At the writing of this book I am proud to be the past chair of the Ethics Commission to the American Occupational Therapy Association. I believe in a compassionate approach to the enforcement of ethical issues. It is imperative that ethics guide members through their career and therefore put an integral part of professional practice in the clinic and in the classroom. As links are being made between education, practice, and research, ethical behavior is ever more important. The centennial vision proposes practice that leads to integrity and increased competence in a global society. The profession will be challenged in the coming years to provide practitioner, educators, and researchers to a society that demands competence and ethical reasoning. This book (Chapter 9) gives some guidelines to the practice of ethics as it relates to spirituality by identifying the principles in the Code of Ethics.

My attempt to bring the philosophy of holism together with an emphasis on spirituality in occupational therapy is a challenge. Nowhere that I know of in the United States does a program in occupational therapy offer a doctoral education with an emphasis on spirituality, nor is there knowledgeable faculty at a doctoral-level programs in occupational therapy who could guide research in spirituality. The existing doctoral programs in religious studies did not meet my specific needs and goals that I personally was looking for at the time. I wanted to continue to conduct research on spirituality in the context of occupational therapy. For me, the answer was to enter into the study of ministry. The course of study in seminary enhanced my knowledge and skills in religious concepts at a scholarly and personal level. It also promoted an interfaith philosophy, which is important in the health care profession. Interfaith and ecumenical philosophy is another theme emphasized throughout this book. Chapter 6 discusses the world's major religions and their possible impact on the clinical setting.

This book is for students, educators, and therapists. I hope it will meet the needs of a profession that is looking for assessment methods and treatment principles to apply in the context of spirituality. The *Occupational Therapy Practice Framework* (AOTA, 2008, 2014) does not suggest how to apply spirituality in the delivery of health care. Many occupational therapists are people of faith and may need guidance in applying spiritual concepts in their treatment settings. I do hope this book may come of some help.

Courses in spirituality need to be developed across curricula, because the therapists of the future should be able to apply spiritual concepts. As students journey through the educational process, they can emerge as professionals who are compassionate and comfortable with their own spirituality, and able to develop the therapeutic use of self, and become skilled in directly applying occupations that will enhance the client's wellness in a truly holistic manner. I further hope that current therapists who are looking for the means to apply spirituality to the clinical setting can, with confidence, relate to their clients on a spiritual level.

Barbara J. Hemphill, DMin, OTR, FAOTA
Doctor of Ministry
Associate Professor Emeritus
Western Michigan University

## References

American Occupational Therapy Association (AOTA). (2008). Occupational therapy practice framework: Domain and process. *American Journal of Occupational Therapy, 56*, 609–639.

American Occupational Therapy Association (AOTA). (2014). Occupational therapy practice framework: Domain and process (2nd ed.). *American Journal of Occupational Therapy, 62*, 625–683.

Christiansen, C., & Baum, C. (Eds.). (1997). *Enabling function and well-being* (2nd ed.). Thorofare, NJ: Slack.

Crepeau, E. B., Cohn, E. S., & Schell, B. A. B. (Eds.). (2003). *Willard and Spackman's occupational therapy.* New York: Lippincott Williams & Wilkins.

Engel, D. (1974). Religion, education and the law. In D. E. Engel (Ed.), *Religion in public education* (pp. 41–51). New York: Paulist Press.

Fowler, J. (1981). *Stages of faith: The psychology of human development and the quest for meaning.* San Francisco: Harper.

Hemphill, B. (1982). *Training manual for the BH battery*, Thorofare, NJ: Slack.

Jacobs, K., & Jacobs, L. (2004). *Quick reference dictionary for occupational therapy* (4th ed.). Thorofare, NJ: Slack.

Moody, H., & Carroll, D. (1997). *The five stages of the soul.* New York: Doubleday.

Mosey, A. (1986). *Psychosocial components of occupational therapy.* New York: Raven Press.

Peck, S. (1987). *The different drum: Community making and peace.* New York: Simon & Schuster.

Peck, S. (1997). *The road less traveled and beyond: Spiritual growth in the age of anxiety.* New York: Simon & Schuster.

Reed, K., & Sanderson, S. (1999). *Concepts of occupational therapy* (4th ed.). Philadelphia: Lippincott Williams & Wilkins.

Siegel, B. (1990). *Love, medicine, and miracles.* New York: Harper & Row.

Wilcock, A. (1989). *An occupational perspective on health.* Thorofare, NJ: Slack.

Wilcock, A. (2006). *An occupational perspective on health* (2nd ed.). Thorofare, NJ: Slack.

Zemke, R., & Clark, F. (1996). *Occupational science: The evolving discipline.* Philadelphia: F. A. Davis.

### *Related reading*

Punwar, A., & Peloquin, S. (2000). *Occupational therapy principles and practice* (3rd ed.). Baltimore: Lippincott Williams & Wilkins.

Swarbrick, P., & Burkhardt, A. (2000). Spiritual health: Implications for the occupational therapy process. *Mental Health Special Interest Section Quarterly, 23*(2), 1–3.

Urbanowski, R., & Vargo, J. (1994). Spirituality, daily practice, and the occupational performance model. *Canadian Journal of Occupational Therapy, 61*, 88–94.

# Acknowledgments

I am appreciative to my mentor Dr. & Rev. Charles Kutz-Marks. Dr. Kutz-Marks is senior minister at the University Christian Church in Austin, Texas. He listened to my goals, my theology, and my passion for my topic. He guided my thinking, helped me express my thoughts, and gave editorial feedback. Dr. Kutz-Marks was instrumental in guiding my thinking about the relationship between occupational therapy and spirituality. He read my manuscript without judgment and with encouragement and gave me valuable input.

To my husband John Pearson, I am forever grateful. John read my project many times for clarity of content, and organization. His influences helped me to clarify my thoughts about spirituality and theology so that it made sense to a non-health care provider.

To Christine Urish who helped develop learning objectives, and suggested resources for each chapter. I am grateful for her skills, talent, and knowledge.

# 1 Introduction

## Theology of occupation

**Chapter objectives**

1  Define theology in the health context.
2  Discuss the Mind, Body, Spirit (Soul) relationship
3  Discuss the development of the ego.

In his book *Way of Blessing, Way of Life*, Williamson (1999), a leading theologian, offered a definition of theology that provides a means for conversation without the traditional "God" language and brings together concepts that do not normally lend themselves to dialogue with each other: theology and occupation. He describes theology as a way of life and as we walk in time that has its ups and downs. He reflected that

> theology is the practical wisdom, the result and process of thinking about matters of faith, that seeks to help us walk the way of faith without straying from the path of the life and blessing or that tries to help find the path again after we have lost it for awhile.
>
> (Williamson, 1999, p. 18)

The practice of talking and communicating with each other through faith has been called *theology*. Theology is an

> ongoing conversation with ourselves, with others, within a … context, and with our tradition. It is not the absolute Truth worked out in solitude from the point of view of someone perched on a mountaintop looking down on all the human beings struggling through the valley below.
>
> (Williamson, 1999, p. 23)

One's theology is expressed in form, function, and meaning in the outer world through occupation.

The science of occupation focuses on three aspects: form, function, and meaning. *Form* means direct observations of occupations, such as practices that express a person's faith tradition. Examples are praying, meditating, and prostrating. These activities and rituals express one's theology about religious faith.

*Function* "refers to the ways occupation influences development, adaptation, health and quality of life" (Larson, Wood, & Clark, 2003, p. 15.) An example of function is how happiness is related to satisfaction in life relative to a faith tradition.

*Meaning* is "the significance of occupation within the context of real lives and in culture" (Larson et al., 2003, p. 16). Examples include the relationship of meaning to self-expression and identity and how meaning influences choice of occupation. Meaning is the subjective experience that happens in occupations; one assigns personal significance and value to occupation. Religious practices that are meaningful to the spirit will be maintained and sustained over time.

## Biology

Developing and maintaining spirituality in the self that is in relation to the outer world involves having a theology. Newberg, D'Aquili, and Rause (2001) hypothesized that "spiritual experience, at its very root, is intimately interwoven with human biology. That biology, in some way, compels the spiritual urge" (p. 8). The limbic system is integral to religious and spiritual experience. In the cerebral cortex, the brain and mind reside and together they create a person's self image and worldview.

## Self, mind

Within the human there is an inner, personal awareness, a free-standing, observant self. Newberg et al. (2001) defined *brain* as a "collection of physical structures that gather and process sensory, cognitive and emotional data: the *mind* is the phenomenon of thoughts, memories, and emotions that arise from the perceptual processes of the brain" (p. 33). The mind could be seen "as something separate from the brain, a free-floating consciousness that could be considered a 'soul'" (p. 34). The self is not the same as the mind; the mind exists before the self and makes possible memories, emotions, affect associated with caring, meaningfulness, and other essential parts of the self.

In other words, this can be viewed as a hierarchy with the brain being the lowest denominator. The mind is at the second order and functions as a result of brain function. The mind is present at birth and the true self (observant self) is derived from the mind. Without the mind, the observant self cannot develop and the individual cannot perceive itself from the outer world. The brain and mind have to function in order to recognize observant self. The soul is the highest order and the mind can be the same as the soul and it is through the observant self that there is a connection with the soul and, therefore, experience spirituality.

Within the cerebral cortex are association areas that correspond to the various regions of the brain. One such area is the orientation association area, which is located near the parietal lobe. It helps distinguish the self from the rest of the world and orients that self in space. If this area loses function, a person is unable to find the boundaries of his or her body, and the mind is no longer able to perceive a sense of self at all. There is no ego. Spirituality includes having a theology about relationships with oneself and others as well as having a world-view that results in the quality of life.

## Occupation and spirituality

What is quality of life to one person may be different to another. Christiansen and Baum (1977) stated that quality of life is defined by the client's perspective of performance in four areas; physical and occupational function, psychological state of mind, social interaction, and somatic or bodily state. Spirituality can be included in any one of those areas. Occupations restore doing in people with disabilities or maintain doing in people who are well. Researchers study what people do in life, and the central tenet of the science of occupation is the idea that people adapt to situations in the environment through occupation. That is, they adapt through deliberate, mindful, organized action. In the life of a spiritual person, it is important to be able to adapt to the environment. Occupational therapy emphasizes adapting while engaging in an activity. The result is quality of life (Zemke & Clark, 1996).

Spiritual quality of life is achieved through relationships that promote inter-connectedness among humans, the world, and a transcendent entity (a higher power)—or, in occupational therapy, among the client, the therapist, and a higher power. Quality of life is "a state of well-being and functioning that includes a level of comfort, enjoyment, and the ability to participate in meaning-ful activities or occupations" (Crepeau, Cohn, & Schell, 2003, p. 1033). Mean-ingfulness in human spirituality happens in the mind (Newberg et al., 2001).

Spirituality is performed in the context of the self and the outer world. Health care services are carried out in the treatment setting and are influenced by the client's beliefs, perceptions, and culture. Spirituality, whether conscious or unconscious, is expressed through action in the world. The client's culture and customs are seated in the external world and influence how services are delivered (American Occupational Therapy Association [AOTA], 2008, 2014).

## Religion, spirituality, and soul

A distinction must be made among religion, spirituality, and soul. Spirituality is definitely a part of religion, but religion may not be a part of spirituality. Spiritu-ality contains the domains of religion but need not adhere to a religious ideo-logy. The understanding of spirituality is often limited by the words that are used to describe it. It includes the aspects of higher consciousness, transcendence, self-reliance, love, faith, enlightenment, community, self-actualization, compas-sion, forgiveness, mysticism, a higher power, grace, and a multitude of other qualities. Sometimes determining what a concept is *not* becomes a method of defining it. For example, spirituality is neither a religion nor the practice of a religion. Human spirituality is not bound by dogma, although it is often associ-ated with religion. Although *spirituality* refers to personal concepts concerning human life, *religiosity* usually relates to more formalized systems of worship that involve beliefs and behaviors shared by others to promote a connection with a divine source.

Seaward (2013) stated that spirituality has three components:

1    The relationship, which is both intrapersonal and interpersonal.
2    One's personal value system.
3    One's purpose to life, referred to as *personal well-being*.

Motivation is essential to wellness and spiritual health. Spirituality is the manifestation of the soul.

Early Western civilization did not separate humans into body, mind, and spirit. The Hebrew understanding of the soul was that it referred to the total person. Aelred Squire (1976) stated, "Man does not have a soul, he is a soul" (p. 19). May (1982) further explained that the fundamental essence of a person is the soul, "while the spirit is the aspect of that essence that gives it power, energy, and motive force" (p. 32). The soul is the inner self, whereas spirituality is the expression of the self in the world. May (1982) continued, "Thus soul and spirit are not 'things' in which one may choose to believe or not to believe. They are simply descriptive aspects of our existence, the one referring to our essence and the other to our fundamental energy" (p. 32). He argued that the mystery of spirit is the search for an "experiential appreciation of the meaning of life"; he believed "that search is a spiritual quest" and that "if followed deeply enough, it will inevitably come upon mystery" (May, 1982, p. 32). According to May, people are born having a soul in perfect form. It remains perfect throughout life. It is irrelevant to this discussion whether the soul is created at conception or birth. The spirit is the manifestation of the soul. Outer forces, such as one's community, culture, social status, and religious tradition shape the spirit.

Parker Palmer (2004) named four functions of the soul:

1    The soul wants to keep us rooted in the ground of our own being, resisting the tendency of other faculties, such as the intellect and ego, to uproot us from who we are.
2    The soul wants to keep us connected to the community in which we find life, for it understands that relationships are necessary if we are to thrive.
3    The soul wants to tell us the truth about ourselves, our world, and the relation between the two, whether that truth is easy or hard to hear.
4    The soul wants to give us life and wants us to pass that gift along, to become life-givers in a world that deals too much in death.

(pp. 33–34)

We go through daily life engaging in occupations that the soul persistently draws us back to—the essence that is connected to the divine. As Palmer (2004) noted,

"Thomas Merton called it true self. Buddhists called it original nature or big self. Hasidic Jews called it the spark of the divine, and humanists called it identity and integrity" (p. 33). In other words, the soul is that which is connected to the divine or the true self. The spirit is the quest for the meaning of life, and the occupations are the forces and motivations that result in sustainable actions. Occupations draw one back to the soul.

A newborn baby's brain recognizes two kinds of sensory input; the "first is input resulting from his behavior, [the] second from behaviors he does not generate or control" (Newburg et al., 2001, p. 150). Newburg et al. (2001) believed that the "perception of these categories is the first step in the brain's inclination to draw a line between the inner reality of the self and the external reality of the world" (p. 150).

Hasselkus (2002) used the metaphor of an inside room and an outside room to address spirituality. The inner room can be likened to the true self—the soul (inner reality of the self)—and the outer room can be likened to the outer self, or the spirit (the reality of the world). The outer self is where the ego resides. The divine inner self is our essence; the outer self contains the spirit. Through spirit, people express their beliefs about health, occupations, and the presence or lack of a higher power. Religious domains, such as values, forgiveness, meaning, and attitudes, are included in the concept of the spirit. The spirit conveys a person's theology. It holds the recognition of the illness experience, the client's faith history, and the story the client has about the illness's effect on the meaning of life. In the spirit is an awareness of one's own spiritual journey and the under-standing of occupation's role in a reciprocal relationship between the spirit and the soul and between the client and the therapist.

Relationships with other people and the world take place in the spiritual self. The relationship among the client, the therapist, and a transcendent being is triadic. Through creative expression in the spirit, the world of doing takes place. Spiritual health requires a balance or congruence between the soul and spirit—a balance among one's physical, mental, and social capacities. One's behavior in the world reflects the soul. When a person has a disease or illness, the soul and spirit are out of balance, and the person's behaviors no longer express his or her spirituality. There is dissonance, and the client is in spiritual distress.

The therapist's goal is to achieve balance through the therapeutic relationship. The relationship between the occupational therapist and the client involves the soul and spirit of both persons. This interaction, in the context of the treatment setting, can be a spiritual experience when each person is receptive to the other's soul and spirit.

Occupation acts like a vehicle through which the soul can communicate with the spirit. For example, a therapist might use the occupation of projective media to help the client express an imbalance between the soul (inner world) and spirit (the outer world). Through painting, the client is able to express this imbalance in the outer world, where it has meaning.

An occupation need not be a ritual or include special objects or symbols to have spiritual meaning. When a person pays particular attention to the way an occupation is done and the context in which it is performed, that occupation becomes an opportunity for meaning. Kabat-Zinn (1994) suggested that any occupation can be an activity of spirit if attention is given to its style and context.

Hasselkus (2002) stated,

> We think of occupation as a vehicle by which our internal world [spiritual self] is expressed in our external world [outer self], i.e., by which our spiritual consciousness is given expression in our daily lives. Occupation opens the door between the inside room and the outside room; occupation unites the internal and external dimensions of our selves.
>
> (p. 112)

In occupational therapy, through meaningful activities, each person's spiritual occupation is expressed through occupational performances in the outer world. For example, church attendance, prayer, other religious activities, congregational support, religious commitment, and religious preferences are in the world of doing and provide a connection between spirituality and the outer world. Not all religious occupation expresses the spiritual self. Rituals or creeds that have religious functions do not necessarily express the spirituality of the individual. Conversely, some occupations that express the spiritual self are not religious. Occupational performances such as meditation, yoga exercises, and imaging could be considered spiritual activities that can be meaningful but are not necessarily associated with religious practice.

In the treatment process, therapists perform the occupations that are specific to the role of a health care provider, including intervention techniques and assessments. Therapists also bring to the treatment setting their own soul and sense of spirituality, which are expressed in their faith traditions. The therapist may be able to achieve a balance between the soul and the spiritual self by using the principles of holism to help move the client from the soul to the spiritual self. Occupation is used to allow the spirit to be expressed in the client's everyday life through form, function, and meaning.

Principles of motivation help sustain occupation. Occupations that are meaningful are internally motivated and are so sustained. The therapist can and may use activities to make conscious that which is unconscious and to help the client express his or her spiritual needs in the outer world. Spiritual activities that have meaning will be repeated and expressed.

The soul of the therapist contains the means by which he or she can connect with the soul of the client. The literature supports the idea that techniques and principles of treatment are not enough for successful treatment and that the self makes a critical difference. The *therapeutic use of self* is a type of ministry that manifests itself in the relationship established between therapist and client during the therapeutic process.

# Summary

The theology of occupation is the belief in the interrelationship between the outer self (world) and the inner self (mind and soul). Theology of occupation is the belief about the interaction between the brain, the mind, and the soul. It is occupation that allows the inner self and the outer self to interact where occupation becomes meaningful. The brain functions to allow the individual to interact with the outer world through creative expressions—it is the world of doing. The brain organ acts on the world through processing sensory, cognitive, and emotional experiences. The brain is the lowest functioning and is responsible for the interaction with the outer self. The mind is the next level and is responsible for the observant self. The observant self then interacts with the soul—the inner self experiences spirituality. The mind is present at birth and the observant self (inner self) is a result of the interaction between the mind and the brain. The ego self (outer self) is also developed out of the mind, but it is a result of interaction between the mind and the outer world. Without this interaction there is no ego. The soul expresses itself through occupation. Another way of looking at it is in the form of a triangle with the brain at its base. In the middle is the mind. The mind is responsible for thoughts, feelings, functioning. The mind houses the observant self. At the pinnacle is the soul. While the brain interacts with the mind, the mind interacts with the soul. It is through this interaction (mind and soul) that a transcendent being (higher power) is realized. The individual is capable of having a spiritual experience with the inner self and the soul. Humans are therefore a soul. The soul functions to resist the trappings of the brain—the intellect and ego. It helps to keep individuals in community, to tell the individual the truth about themselves, and tries to have an effect on the world around.

Spirituality as an occupation provides a pathway between the outer world and the inner world of the self. It is a means by which to return to the true self and connection with the divine. The spirit resides between the inner self and the outer self. And it is the spirit that gives expression of the inner self to the outer world. Individuals express their spirituality, their values, their beliefs about illness and health, and their faith tradition in occupation. It is through occupation that individuals tell their story about illness experiences, and their meaning in life.

In the therapeutic environment, the therapist performs the occupation consistent with a health care provider. The client and therapist have a reciprocal relationship in which each expresses the inner self of the soul. The spirituality of each is expressed through occupation. The next chapter will go into greater detail of the relationship between spirituality and occupational therapy.

This chapter presents a definition of theology; discusses the relationship between occupation and spirituality; describes the theology of occupation; and presents a scheme for understanding the relationship among soul, spirituality, and occupation. It makes the following points:

- Developing and maintaining spirituality in the self in relation to the outer world involves having a theology.

- Spirituality is performed in the context of the self and the outer world.
- Spirituality is the manifestation of the soul.
- The soul is the inner self, whereas spirituality is the expression of the self in the world.
- The soul is that which is connected to the divine or the true self. The spirit is the quest for the meaning of life, and occupations are the forces and motivations that result in sustainable actions. Occupations draw the person back to the soul.
- The inner self is the true self.
- The outer self is where the ego resides, and the inner self is a person's essence.
- The outer self contains the spirit.
- Through spirit, beliefs about health and occupations are expressed.
- Occupations act as a vehicle so that the soul can communicate with the spirit.
- Occupations allow passage between the inner self and the outer self.
- Through meaningful activities such as church attendance, prayer, and religious practices, each person's spiritual occupation is expressed in the outer world.

**Active learning strategies**

1   Write a personal paper about the relationship between mind, body, and spirit.
2   Write a personal theology paper about the relationship between spirituality and occupation.

**References**

American Occupational Therapy Association (AOTA). (2008). Occupational therapy practice framework: Domain and process. *American Journal of Occupational Therapy, 56*, 609–639.

American Occupational Therapy Association (AOTA). (2014). Occupational therapy practice framework: Domain and process (2nd ed.). *American Journal of Occupational Therapy, 62*, 625–683.

Christiansen, C., & Baum, C. (Eds.). (1997). *Enabling function and well-being* (2nd ed.). Thorofare, NJ: Slack.

Crepeau, E. B., Cohn, E., & Schell, B. A. B. (2003). *Willard and Spackman's occupational therapy* (10th ed., p. 1033). Philadelphia: Lippincott Williams & Wilkins.

Hasselkus, B. (2002). *The meaning of everyday occupation.* Thorofare, NJ: Slack.

Kabat-Zinn, J. (1994). *Wherever you go, there you are: Mindfulness meditation in everyday life.* New York: Hyperion.

Larson, E., Wood, W., & Clark, F. (2003). Occupational science: Building the science and practice of occupation through an academic discipline. In E. Crepeau, E. Cohn, & B. Schell (Eds.), *Willard and Spackman's occupational therapy* (pp. 15–24). New York: Lippincott Williams & Wilkins.

May, G. (1982). *Will and spirit: A contemplative psychology.* New York: HarperCollins.

Meyer, A. (1922). Philosophy of occupational therapy. *Archives of Occupational Therapy, 1,* 1–10.

Newberg, A., D'Aquili, E., & Rause, V. (2001). *Why God won't go away.* New York: Ballantine.

Palmer, P. (2004). *A hidden wholeness: The journey toward an undivided life.* San Francisco: Jossey-Bass.

Seaward, B. (2013). *Health of the human spirit: Spiritual dimensions for personal health* (2nd ed.). London: Johns & Bartlett Learning.

Squire, A. (1976). *Asking the fathers* (2nd ed.). Wilton, CT: Morehouse-Barlow.

Williamson, C. (1999). *Way of blessing, way of life: A Christian theology.* St. Louis, MO: Chalice Press.

Zemke, R., & Clark, F. (1996). *Occupational science: The evolving discipline.* Philadelphia: F. A. Davis.

# 2 Spirituality and occupational therapy

## Chapter objectives

1 Reader will be able to discern the difference between spirituality and religion.
2 Identify statistics related to identification of spirituality versus religiousness.

Spirituality is often associated with religion. Although *spirituality* refers to a personal meaning concerning human life, *religiosity* usually relates to more formalized systems of worship, with beliefs and behaviors shared by others to promote spiritual connection with a divine source. The two tend to occur together. People who say they are spiritual do not necessarily have to hold religious beliefs. Religion is one way in which a person may choose to express or enhance spirituality, but not every spiritual person is religious.

## Lay literature

In 1988, *Better Homes and Gardens* published a questionnaire about spirituality (Greer, 1988). The 80,000 respondents, who included Protestants, Catholics, and Jews, among other faiths, submitted definitions of spirituality. One respondent, for example, separated religion from spirituality by stating,

> Spirituality, in our society, is inappropriately linked to religion. Certainly morality and religious belief do not necessarily agree. Tolerance, consideration, and humanitarianism have little to do with a belief in God. Spirituality is not morality and cannot be practiced by the unbeliever.
>
> (Greer, 1988, p. 25)

The *Better Homes and Gardens* article (Greer, 1988) summarized that spirituality is not the same as morality but that one must have a sense of something beyond oneself to be a believer. Religion is observable, whereas spirituality is less so. Another questionnaire respondent commented on the inadequacy of differentiating between spirituality and religion, and other readers agreed; 74% of the respondents answered *yes* to the question "Is it possible to be a moral, ethical person without being spiritual?" Spirituality has more to do with relationships with a higher being, the self, and other beings than with morality.

Another respondent addressed the concept of motivation in spirituality: "Spiritual strength will motivate the individual to search in depth for an answer to questions of eternity and continuity. This may involve a religious institution, but is not dependent on it" (Greer, 1988, p. 26). The concept of motivation is important, because without motivation a person does not seek a spiritual life or engage in a meaningful activity. Motivation is an essential ingredient in patient wellness and spiritual health. One respondent stated,

> Religion is going through the motions, while faith and trust in God is an experience of the heart. My faith in God is the very core of what I am. It holds my life together through good times and bad.
>
> (Greer, 1988, p. 26)

This respondent expressed the religious concept of spirituality as a measure of faith. Nevertheless, when asked, "Is it possible to be a spiritual person without being religious?" 52% of the respondents answered *yes.* This was a higher number than expected by the researchers.

*Newsweek* conducted a survey where subscribers were asked to send in their response to questions about spirituality (Adler, 2005). The survey found that 79% of 10,004 respondents described themselves as "spiritual," whereas 64% said they were "religious." Fifty-five percent of the respondents reported that they were religious and spiritual, and 24% reported that they were spiritual but not religious. Sixty-four percent said they prayed, 29% meditated, 21% participated in a spiritual activity not connected with church, 20% read the Bible or Koran, and only 2% attended church or other services. In addition, 20% had changed faiths since childhood, and 4% had abandoned religion altogether.

The *Better Homes and Gardens* (Greer, 1988) and *Newsweek* (Adler, 2005) articles do not present data obtained through a controlled scientific study. They were national surveys, however, and the data may represent the population being admitted into medical facilities and finding their way to occupational therapy clinics. Most people who responded to the *Newsweek* poll said they were spiritual (57% said that spirituality was very important in their daily life) but not religious, and a small number said they were unchurched (not attending any kind of worship service on a regular basis). One-third said they were evangelical Protestant, but the other two-thirds said they were other Christian denominations, Jewish, Muslim, or atheist.

Religiosity connotes belonging to and practicing a religious tradition. Larson, Wood, and Clark (2003) identified it as "form" in occupation; it includes activities that are directly associated with a religious tradition, such as taking communion, praying at certain times of the day, or meditating. The religious person engages in meaningful occupation that expresses his or her theology. Religious theology is associated with the function of spirituality; it influences development of spirituality and promotes quality of life and health. Being spiritual is a personal commitment to a process of inner development that engages the person's totality (a person's quality, i.e., the well-being of the whole person, desirable or undesirable). Spiritual occupations are not obvious and are undertaken in the context of culture, ethnicity, and race. Religion is one way of expressing spirituality. Not every religious person is spiritual, and not every spiritual person is religious. If spirituality is to add meaning to life and improve quality of life, a person's religious activities can fill the function of a spiritual occupation. In the practice of a religious tradition or a spiritual occupation, form, function, and meaning can be considered occupations.

The occupational therapy literature addresses spiritual concepts. The therapist should try to recognize whether the client relates to spirituality through a religious discipline or by other methods and should assist the client in his or her spiritual process if the client desires. A religious therapist, however, may be uncomfortable with unconventional spirituality. Peloquin (2003) offered the following concepts that are spiritual but do not imply religiosity:

- Belief in a transcendent dimension to life
- Belief in some meaning and purpose to life
- Belief in a sense of personal mission
- Belief that life is infused with sacredness
- Belief that material values are of themselves insufficient
- Altruism
- Idealism
- Awareness of the tragic realities of human existence
- Awareness that a spiritual sense is fruitful.

(p. 122)

These concepts imply that many people have a spiritual life without being religious. Spiritual matters become important when people seek assistance from occupational therapists.

> According to our *Code of Ethics* [American Occupational Therapy Association] and medical ethicists we are morally obliged to act in certain ways that reflect what it means to be professional, to respond to fellow human beings who place trust in us because of their vulnerability in time of need.
>
> (Davis, 1997, p. 9)

## Definition of spirituality from the occupational therapy literature

In the occupational therapy literature, McColl (2003) defined spirituality as "sensitivity to the presence of spirit" (p. 244). From a theological perspective, spirit is shared among humans. McColl (1998) noted that whereas spirituality is a human characteristic, spirit is not. Spirit is ... independent of [humans] and can be incorporated into ... lives to a greater and lesser extent, depending on the extent to which ... [one is] able to experience it—that is, depending on the extent of [one's] spirituality.

(p. 244)

The theological literature suggests that one experiences the spirit through a transcendent being. Because there is no occupational therapy language to express the experience of the transcendent being, the use of occupation is part of the spiritual expression.

McColl (2003) further identified four themes in the occupational therapy literature that address spirituality:

1   Spirituality entails an innate knowledge of the essence of the self.
2   It is the source of our will, intention, and self-determination.
3   It is responsible for the connection among people.
4   It invests our daily occupation with meaning.

(p. 245)

McColl (2003) added that spirituality includes the concepts of the divine self, the intentionality of the spirit, and the relationship with other people. It supports the triadic relationship among the divine, the self, and others, which includes activities that are meaningful to the soul. According to McColl (2003), occupations become meaningful when they reach the soul.

Pierce (2003) offered another definition of spirituality. She stated that "spirituality is a source of energy that comes from inner beliefs about life's meaning. For some ... spirituality is a set of activities existing within the framework of a religious community" (p. 170). For example, people of faith may gather for worship and to study, pray, and observe holidays. Spirituality may consist of occupational performances that express the person's beliefs about a transcendent being. Some people, however, engage in activities such as meditation and study groups without belonging to any specific religion. It is important for therapists to understand that some religious activities are not spiritual and that some activities that do not seem spiritual are so to a particular person. A definition of spirituality in occupational therapy needs to reflect this understanding.

The occupational therapy literature that addresses spirituality states that it is associated with the meaning of life and escapes the conscious awareness of most people. As a result, people who are on a spiritual journey may not be aware of this journey during their daily life. Spirituality has a subjective nature, but it becomes clear to a person in the context of life activities. Urbanowski and Vargo (1994) stated that it is reasonable to assume that people "develop a conscious awareness of the meaning of life within the context of the activities of their daily lives" and that spirituality is viewed as "the experience of meaning in everyday life activities" (p. 6). Becoming aware of one's spirituality through experiences one has when engaged in activities is a sign of a mature spiritual journey.

Occupational therapy is concerned with people's ability to perform occupations. Its goal is to help people independently fulfill roles and perform or control the performance of meaningful activities. Collins, Stanley, and West-Frasier (2001) suggested that spirituality is the experience of meaning within a person. This definition implies that any activity that has meaning to a person has the potential to express spirituality (Collins et al., 2001).

The Canadian Association of Occupational Therapists ([CAOT], 1991) has recognized spirituality as an integral component of occupational performance in client-centered practice. The association considers spirituality as one of four components necessary for a holistic view of humans (the other holistic components are mental, physical, and socio-cultural (CAOT, 1991). The inclusion of a spiritual dimension acknowledges a person's sense of self and his or her beliefs about power, control, and meaning in life, because these beliefs are formed internally and are influenced by environmental forces. The Canadian model does not distinguish between religious activities and spiritual activities.

Many occupational therapists use the Canadian model. American therapists, however, are still debating whether spirituality should be a component in their practice. The field has made no effort to distinguish between religious and spiritual activities in any of its official documents, nor has it defined spirituality. American occupational therapy practice (i.e., *Occupation Therapy Practice Framework*; American Occupational Therapy Association [AOTA], 2008) emphasizes the concept of spirituality in context and seems to assume that spirituality and religion are the same. *Spirituality in context* means as it relates to culture, ethnicity, and race, not to occupation.

Occupational therapists, however, do not seem to always agree on how spirituality should be integrated into treatment. To consider it a performance component it is not consistent with the current *Occupational Therapy Practice Framework* (AOTA, 2014). When spirituality is made a performance component instead of client factors, the therapist sees the client as a disability rather than as a person. The therapist may then overemphasize the need to fix the problem and rely overmuch on methods and principles of treatment. He or she may focus on the form of the occupation of spirituality—that is, what can be directly observed. This approach leaves out how spirituality influences development, adaptation, and health. In addition, the field's definition of spirituality does not take into consideration spiritual health. *Spiritual health* (Swarbrick & Burkhardt, 2000) and *spirituality* are overlapping terms. Spirituality is an inner perception and source of strength that are reflected through one's being, knowing, and doing. The meaning of spirituality is not included in the definition of spiritual health. It does not show that spirituality involves a belief in a unifying force, or higher power, that gives meaning and purpose to life and can provide a sense of belonging to something greater than mere existence (Swarbrick & Burkhardt, 2000). Spiritual health is the recognition and ability to put in practice moral and religious beliefs. Emphasis is put on a healthy balance between the mind, body, and spirit.

The term *spiritual* can be defined as the here-and-now experience of meaning in everyday life activities, and it represents the experience of the whole person in that context. It can be looked at as relating to or consisting of the spirit. This experience may be in a context of occupation, consciousness or unconsciousness, conventionality or unconventionality. The Canadian definition does not take into consideration the three factors that facilitate spirituality: awareness, connectedness, and living in the present (Spector, 1996). *Awareness* requires the therapist to listen to and hear the client's illness experience. *Connectedness* involves the self, the self with others, and the community. *Living in the present* means that spiritual experience takes place in the present moment. Meaning does not rest in the past or the future. The past implies something that should have been; the future implies what should be or where a person should be. Spector (1996) stated that the "only place a person can really find meaning is in the experience of here and now" (p. 24).

## Meaningfulness and spirituality

An essential component of spirituality is the concept of meaningfulness. The formulation of a self-identity during adulthood includes appreciating one's life and deriving meaning from it. *Spiritual meaning* refers to a person's sense of self and beliefs about power, control, and meaning in life.

Newberg, D'Aquili, and Rause (2001) stated that how the self is derived is a mystery, but they believed that it arises through a process of reification, which is

the ability to convert a concept into a concrete thing, or ... to bestow upon something the quality of being real or true. In its neurological definition, the term refers to the power of the mind to grant meaning and substance to its own perceptions, thoughts, and beliefs, and to regard them as meaningful.

(p. 149)

McColl (2003) addressed spirituality in the context of meaningfulness:

Not only does spirituality invest activities with meaning, but also meaningful activities express spirituality. [It is important to] distinguish between meaning IN life ... referring to specific activities and the meanings they carry, and the meaning OF life ... referring to the meaning of one's whole life.

(p. 246)

McColl further asserted that opportunities for experiencing transcendence arise every day through activities and that occupations provide connection to the transcendent being and therefore help people derive meaning from those occupations.

Trombly (1995) noted that occupation as an end is meaningful because the person doing an activity views it as important: "Only meaningful occupation remains in the person's life repertoire" (p. 963). Meaningfulness is based on the person's beliefs and values, which are grounded in family and culture. It also depends on the person's sense of what is important. Thus, the person determines the meaningfulness of any occupation as an end. As Reed and Sanderson (1999) noted, "meaningfulness is strongly associated with motivation" (p. 267), and motivation sustains the occupation.

Jung (1933/1957) defined *spirit* as the guiding principle in psychic life; spirit regulates thoughts and allows meaningful insights and a sense of well-being. Therefore, meaning comes from the spirit or the spiritual self. Meaningfulness in the context of activity is born of experiences that have an internal locus or internal self. It comes from within a person who has a spiritual experience while engaging in activity. The spiritual experience is not always conscious, but it can become conscious while the person is immersed in activity. When this happens, it makes activity meaningful and makes contact with the inner soul possible.

Not all activity is meaningful, however, just as spirituality does not always mean religiosity. A person may engage in a religious activity and not be spiritual. Similarly, a person may participate in activities to achieve a goal, but those activities do not necessarily assume a place of central importance or meaning for the person. Howard and Howard (1997) stated, "The central element of religion is the provision of ultimate meaning. Religion allows people to interpret events and experiences as ultimately meaningful by linking them with a larger sense of order" (p. 182).

Also, meaningfulness may or may not include a belief in an internal or external higher power. A person can be an atheist and be a spiritual being because life holds meaning. In the theology of occupation, meaning is a gateway to the soul—the divine self. The inner self is never absent. A spiritual dimension is included in a person's life when he or she acknowledges the sense of self—spiritual self—and beliefs about meaning in life, because these are formed internally. When the therapist is successful, achievement of spiritual health is influenced by the development of a sense of meaning and purpose, a sense of connectedness with the self and others, and one's acceptance of a greater purpose of reality.

Urbanowski and Vargo (1994) defined spirituality as "the experience of meaning in everyday life activities" (p. 91). It seems important to distinguish between "the meaning of life" and "meaning in life." The meaning of life is the "big picture"; it means asking questions about the purpose of living about which a person does not really worry in everyday life. Meaning in life is what people are concerned about in their daily life and activities. As a result, the here-and-now experience resides in the spiritual phenomenon.

The framework from which spirituality is integrated into the practice of occupation comes from a holistic dimension. *Holism* can be defined as a belief in the interactive effects of mind, body, spirit, and environment; the existence of functional interdependence among parts and wholes; and the idea of individual responsibility (Peters, 1991). In practice, holism should be integrated into the treatment plan, which is shared with significant persons, such as family and other health care practitioners. The client is viewed as autonomous and as a coparticipant in health care delivery (White, 1986). Particular attention is paid to biological, psychological, social, spiritual, and environment factors.

The English word *health* is based on the Anglo-Saxon word *hale*, meaning "whole," so to be healthy is to be whole. The word *holy* comes from the same root (Peters, 1991). Humans have always considered wholeness to be an absolute necessity to make life worth living. The relationship between body and soul has been addressed since ancient times. Greek philosophers, biblical writers, and theologians have written about the wholeness of humankind.

## Summary

This chapter has continued to explore the distinction between religion and spirituality. Even though religion is associated with spirituality, the therapist meets the spiritual person in clinic, not the religious person. Definitions have been offered, but none seems to address the person who is not religious but spiritual. The spiritual person has a soul, and meaningful activities that express that soul are occupations—as described in Chapter 1. The Canadian model does not solve the problem of function and does not address the meaningfulness of a spiritual activity. The next chapter discusses the theology of body and soul.

## Active learning strategies

1  See Web Resources below.
2  How do you personally define religion, spirituality? How do the beliefs you hold differ or are similar to those expressed in the text? How do your spiritual beliefs and values guide you as an individual? As a therapist? Begin a reflective journal that you can add to as you work your way through this text.
3  If you were to graphically represent or draw, paint, sketch, create yourself as a spiritual being, what would you look like? If you could choose a symbol, what would it be? Take time to explore your creative spiritual self.
4  Review the *Occupational Therapy Practice Framework* (AOTA, 2014). Create a concept map of where spirituality exists within the Occupational Therapy Practice Framework and how this relates to the patient/client. Many concept map generators are available online.
5  Select an activity that is very meaningful to you as an individual. How does engaging in this activity contribute to your spirituality?

## Web resources

Develop a personal mission statement. There are several books and online resources to assist with this process. A mission statement is often a start to assist an individual in gaining clarity regarding their current situation.

See www.missionstatements.com/personal_mission_statements.html.

# References

Adler, J. (2005, September 5). In search of the spiritual. *Newsweek, 146*(9), 46–64.

American Occupational Therapy Association (AOTA). (2008). Occupational therapy practice framework: Domain and process (2nd ed.). *American Journal of Occupational Therapy, 62*, 625–683.

American Occupational Therapy Association (AOTA). (2014). *Occupational therapy practice framework: Domain and process* (3rd ed.). Bethesda, MD: AOTA Press.

Canadian Association of Occupational Therapists (CAOT). (1991). *Occupational therapy guidelines for client-centered practice.* Toronto, ON: CAOT Publications ACE.

Collins, J., Stanley, P., & West-Frasier, J. (2001). The utilization of spirituality in occupational therapy: Beliefs, practices, and perceived barriers. *Occupational Therapy in Health Care, 14*(3/4), 73–92.

Davis, C. (1997). *Complementary therapies in rehabilitation: Holistic approaches for prevention and wellness.* Thorofare, NJ: Slack.

Greer, K. (1988, January). Special report: Are American families finding new strength in spirituality? *Better Homes and Gardens, 16*(1), 16–27.

Howard, B., & Howard, J. (1997). Occupation as spiritual activity. *American Journal of Occupational Therapy, 51*(3), 181–185.

Jung, C. (1957). *Modern man in search of a soul* (W. S. Dell & C. Baynes, Trans.). New York: Harvest. (Original work published 1933)

Larson, E., Wood, W., & Clark, F. (2003). Occupational science: Building the science and practice of occupation through an academic discipline. In E. Crepeau, E. Cohn, & B. Schell (Eds.), *Willard and Spackman's occupational therapy* (pp. 15–24). Baltimore: Lippincott Williams & Wilkins.

McColl, M. (2003). Spirit, occupation and disability. In R. P. Fleming Cottrell (Ed.), *Perspectives for occupation-based practice* (pp. 243–253). Bethesda, MD: AOTA Press.

Newberg, A., D'Aquili, E., & Rause, V. (2001) *Why God won't go away.* New York: Ballantine.

Peloquin, S. (2003). Spirituality: Meaning related to occupational therapy. In E. Crepeau, E. Cohn, & B. Schell (Eds.), *Willard and Spackman's occupational therapy* (pp. 121–125). Baltimore: Lippincott Williams & Wilkins.

Peters, T. (1991). *The cosmic self.* San Francisco: HarperCollins.

Pierce, D. (2003). *Occupation by design.* New York: F. A. Davis.

Reed, K., & Sanderson, S. (1999). *Concepts of occupational therapy* (4th ed.). Philadelphia: Lippincott Williams & Wilkins.

Spector, M. (1996, May). Developing therapeutic use of self through spirituality. *Journal of Occupational Therapy Students*, 21–26.

Swarbrick, P., & Burkhardt, A. (2000). Spiritual health: Implications for the occupational therapy process. *Mental Health Special Interest Section Quarterly, 23*(2), 1–3.

Trombly, C. A. (1995). Purposefulness and meaningfulness as therapeutic mechanism. 1995 Eleanor Clark Slagle Lecture. *American Journal of Occupational Therapy, 49*, 960–972.

Urbanowski, R., & Vargo, J. (1994). Spirituality, daily practice, and the occupational performance model. *Canadian Journal of Occupational Therapy, 61*(2), 88–94.

White, V. (1986). Promoting health and wellness: A theme for the eighties. *American Journal of Occupational Therapy, 40*, 745–748.

# 3   Theology of body and soul

## Chapter objectives

1   Origin of the terminology, with various definitions and usages. This section includes the traditions of Hinduism, Buddhism, Islam, Christianity, and Judaism.
2   A discussion of the Greek philosophers who addressed body and soul in ancient writings, followed by views of theologians from ancient times.
3   How the terms *body* and *soul* were used in the Old and New Testaments of the Bible, including the Judaic usage.
4   Application of this information to occupational therapy.

References to Christian scripture are given in accordance with the verse and chapter divisions of the New Revised Standard Version of the Bible.

## Origin and definition of *body* and *soul*

The origin and definition of *body* and *soul* come from a variety of worldviews. Pagels (1997) stated that Greek philosophers and Hindu and Buddhist traditions viewed that spirit as the essence of the person that resides in the body. According to Smith (1991), the basic theological concepts of Islam are virtually identical to those of Judaism and Christianity. In the Islamic perspective, the intellect and the spirit are closely related and are two faces of the same reality. In the Islamic tradition, it is important to know the self, and within the self is the divine God—the soul. The Koran states, "And we shall show you our signs to the horizons and in yourselves—do you not see?" (Sura 41:53). This verse is interpreted as God's order to look into one's own heart to find the source of knowledge and, eventually, the divine beloved, who is "closer than the jugular vein" (Sura 50:16). On the basis of this statement, Schimmel (1975) wrote that "who knows himself knows his lord" (p. 189). Drawing on this tradition, one could say that to know one's innermost heart means to discover the point at which the divine is found. The heart is where God resides.

The Koran addresses the relationship between the body and soul. Islamic tradition affirms God through destruction of the body rather than construction.

This means that the body has to be broken and the heart, too, has to be broken so that God can build a new mansion for Himself in it. "For the ruined house contains treasures," Schimmel (1975) wrote; "such treasures can only be found by digging up the foundation" (p. 190).

The Koran presents two doctrines—one about the human self, and the other about the Day of Judgment—that define the soul. These doctrines center on the soul's individuality and freedom. In contrast to the "no self" of Buddhism and the social self of Confucianism, the Koran stresses the self's individuality. As Smith (1991) stated, "All life is individual; there is no such thing as universal life. God Himself is an individual; He is the most unique individual. The individual soul is everlasting, for once it is created, it never dies" (p. 240). In some respects, the theology of the soul in the Islamic tradition is similar to that of the Christian and Jewish traditions. Accordingly, the rest of this discussion focuses on those traditions.

## Definition of terms

*Soma* is a Greek word meaning "body." According to Ferguson (1990), the word was first used by Homer to pertain to a dead human or animal body. Greek thought distinguished the body from the "life-giving breath," or what the philosophers would call "soul." The Greeks saw the body as coextensive with physical existence, but they identified the self as the soul. The body became a symbol of holism. In Greek thought, the body consisted of integrated and organized functions and was governed and directed by the soul. This relationship of body and soul provided a political symbol for the city-state, in which the rulers governed the body politic, just as the soul governed the body. By the 5th century BCE, the term *soma* denoted the trunk or the whole body. The body could be viewed impersonally, but it could also denote the person. Its limitation was that the physical existence ended with death. The body was seen as distinct from the soul, without which it had no value. Physical existence was felt to be an affliction; the body was the *soma* (tomb) of the soul.

The Greek word *psuche* (Latin *anima*), often simply transliterated into English as *psyche* and translated as *soul*, is the nonphysical aspect of life. The soul is a Greek idea. In Homer, the soul was a vague and shadowy concept. The *psuche* denoted a personality that existed before and after the present bodily life; the soul was distinct from and entered the body. In Homeric Greek, *soul* referred to the life principle associated with breath (Hebrew *nephesh*), which departed the body at death "across the teeth's barrier" (Homer 1984, p. 9.409) and led an isolated, insubstantial, and unconscious existence in Hades.

At the end of the 6th century BCE, in Orphic and Pythagorean[1] circles, the belief that a person might be rewarded or punished after death became central, and the term *psuche* was used to denote the essential human "self." *Psuche* referred to the spiritual side of human existence. It indicated both the life principle that animated the body and individuality of the person as expressed in thought, will, and emotion. The soul was the seat of human activity and the source of moral judgment (Hunter, 1990).

Through the distinction between *psyche* and *psuche*, the Greeks understood soul and body. In Orphic sources, the body was described as the soul's tomb (Ferguson, 1990). The dualism of body and soul gave Orphism an ascetic flair that had not characterized Greek life. Asceticism liberated the soul from the impurity of the body, thus serving as the basis for the prohibition of eating animal flesh. According to Ferguson (1993), "in Homer, the living body is the person, and the soul has no prehistory and only a shadowy repetition in the afterlife" (p. 57).

The word *soul* had a very different meaning for the biblical writers. The Hebrew word *nephesh* basically means "breath, " and the term was often used to designate " a living being" (not always a human, sometimes an animal); the word along with the New Testament equivalent, *psyche*, means "life" and even "person" or "self." The term had a broader biblical usage. It stood for the unity of personality, as Hebraic thought saw the human being as a unity rather than as a duality of body and soul.

One can further explain the meaning of *soul* by noting its relationship to the word *body*. Musser and Price (1992) wrote that

> In Pauline thought … body (*soma*) is an exclusive word for the psycho-physical unity of the flesh (*sarx*) and the soul (*psyche*). No hard and fast distinction between the two can be established. The body is the whole person, not a detachable part of a person to be distinguished in dualistic fashion from the soul.
>
> (p. 457)

## The same idea of unity pervaded the Hebrew scriptures

The scriptural view of human nature pointed away from a radical body—soul dualism toward psychosomatic unity. The human was seen as a creature of polarities; the imagery of the Old Testament described clay animated by "breath" (*ruah*) and termed the nonphysical pole of humanity "spirit" (*nephesh*). The *nephesh* was described as descending to Sheol, or Hades, on the death of a person. The term *nephesh* was later extended to the whole person. The Old Testament presented humans as animated beings; it contained a holistic view but also a sense of physical–spiritual polarity, as in Ezekiel 37, where bones and flesh came together but lived only when the animating *ruah* came upon them. *Ruah* indicated the animating principle, and *nephesh* was the animated being (Hunter, 1990).

*Trichotomists* believed that the essential nature of humans had a third part; a spirit that related directly to God (Grudem, 1994). The trichotomists believed that man's soul included the intellect, the emotions, and the will and that all people had this kind of soul, which could either serve God or yield to sin. The trichotomists argued that spirit was a higher faculty that came alive when a person became a Christian. According to Romans 8:10, "if Christ is in you, although your bodies are dead because of sin, your spirits are alive because of righteousness."

## Philosophers' view of body and soul

The Greek philosophers influenced the interpretation of the scriptures, particularly the New Testament, and how the theologians up to the 15th century developed religious doctrine. This chapter reviews the thoughts of the Greek philosophers and ancient theologians who developed the religious doctrine about body and soul. In addition, this chapter reviews holism, an ancient concept that has influenced thinking about occupational therapy.

### Homer (800 BCE)

The *Iliad* opens with a reference to souls (*psychai*) that were hurled down to Hades (Homer, 1984). For Homer, the soul was not one's personality or real self, nor was it the organ of will, intelligence, or desires. It was associated with breath, making the body inactive when it left; the body was nothing but a physical shell. Homer described the soul as having the same height, build, and other characteristics of the body, so that it was recognizable but not embraceable. Death meant passing into a mere shadow of existence, in which the soul could do no more than engage in a reflection of its earthly activities (Ferguson, 1993). Proper burial was very important to Homer. He had a notion of an afterlife—he believed that if a person did not have a proper burial, the soul would wander around, with no place to go.

### Socrates (469–399 BCE)

Socrates was best known for standing in the courtyard giving orations. No actual written manuscripts of his view exist. Eventually, his orations were transcribed by his student, subsequent philosopher, Plato. Socrates tried to get people to give as much attention to their souls as they did to their bodies. By his time, the *psyche* was definitely recognized as the human personality (Ferguson, 1993). Plato's writings represent Socrates' attitude and argument. When Socrates gave his orations in the courtyard, which was the center of where his speeches took place, they were too long at the time to be transcribed or written down.

### Plato (429–347 BCE)

Of all the ancient philosophers, Plato had the greatest influence on the early development of Christian thought. Among Plato's teachings were the doctrines of two worlds, immortality, the preexistence of the soul, knowledge of reminiscence, transmigration of the soul, and the idea of good (Gonzalez, 1970). Plato demonstrated that material things were not ultimate realities. He made an ethical distinction between two worlds, in which the visible world was the homeland of evil, whereas the world of ideas was the goal of human life and morality. From earliest times, the doctrine of immortality of the soul attracted Christians who were searching in Greek philosophy for support for the Christian doctrine of the after-life. The Platonic system made the after-life not a gift of God but the natural result of the divine in the human. Platonic teaching affirmed the eternal life of the soul and the eternal death of the body, because only the spiritual could have permanence (Cullmann, 1958).

## Knowledge of reminiscence

Ferguson (1993) stated that the Platonic theory of knowledge was related to Plato's view of the soul. This view held that people could have concepts only because those concepts were previously known. Ideas were, a priori, known independently of experience. The soul saw and learned ideas before it came into the body. Experience reminded, but it did not prove or validate. The body's senses had the ability to supply information only about objects of the world, not about ideas. Because true knowledge could only be knowledge of ideas, the senses were not an adequate means of attaining knowledge.

Cullmann (1958) stated that Plato used the theory of recall, or *reminiscence*, which required the doctrine and therefore could not interpret knowledge as reminiscent. They did accept the Platonic distrust of sensory perception, however, and through the influence of Augustine, this distrust dominated Christian thought for many centuries.

Plato spoke of three parts of the soul or mind. In *Timaeus and Critias* (Plato, 1977), he specifically described three parts of the soul, which were located in different parts of the body. The powers of reason and decision were situated in the head, which constituted the divine and immortal part of the soul. The head was like the world (or soul), which had its circles of same and different that enabled it to make the basic types of judgment, affirmation, and negation leading to rational thought. In *Timaeus and Critias*, Plato asserted that human souls at their creation were told that any failure in their first incarnation as man would lead to reincarnation as a woman or a lower animal.

The two other parts of the soul, according to Plato, were located in the heart and belly and were mortal. These parts comprised the emotions and feelings, on one hand, and appetite, on the other. These parts of the soul were connected with the physiological processes of the body parts where they were situated. Plato spoke about sensations but little about the "nervous system" (1977, p. 17), although he saw the head as the seat of intelligence. The philosopher made the connection between body and mind and thus between mental and physical disease.

## Transmigration of the soul

In *Timaeus and Critias*, Plato described how the *Demiurge*, or world architect, endowed the world with a soul, the cause of motion, beauty, order, and harmony. This *world soul* was situated between the world of ideas and the world of things that were seen and experienced. The physical world acted according to laws— the laws of its own nature—and was the cause of all law; harmony; and order of life, mind, and knowledge. The soul was the principle of life; it moved the stars, so all the stars had a soul; and it moved the animals and plants, so animals and plants also had souls. The "world soul" also moved bodies, so humans had souls, and it moved the whole universe, so there was a world soul (Ferguson, 1990). According to Tillich (1968), "this soul-principle … is the productive power of the existing world; it forms and controls matter, as our life-principle forms and controls every cell in our body" (p. 52).

The *Demiurge* created souls for all of the planets and all individual souls. These individual souls were eternal, having existed before they came into bodies. In this preexistence, each soul saw all pure ideas in a realm of perfect ideas. The body clouded the soul and forgot all that it had seen. Frost (1962) wrote that "the soul is pulled down and debased by the body" (p. 157). Thus, the goal of the soul was to free itself from the body so that it could see truth. Through experiences, the soul recalled the pure ideas that it viewed in its preexistent state. Knowledge was not new to the soul but was remembrance of what was forgotten because of the body. The human soul was a part of the reason; it existed before it came into the body and, after the body had been destroyed, freed itself from the body and continued to exist. The soul, for Plato, was immortal.

Plato offered several "proofs" of the immortality of the human soul: (1) the soul was in the simplest form and could not be divided or destroyed; (2) the soul was life, and it was not possible that life could become not-life—neither could it become the other (Frost, 1962).

### Aristotle (384–322 BCE)

Aristotle saw himself as the successor of Plato. Aristotle preferred to speak of powers of soul rather than parts of the soul. He believed that three kinds of souls existed:

1    Nutritive or vegetative souls were the lowest souls. They possessed the principles of life, nutrition, repair, and reproduction.
2    Sensitive or animal souls, besides possessing the principles of life, possessed sensations, impulses and instincts. The sensitive souls were the source of desire and motion, which separated animal life from plant life.
3    Thinking or rational souls, the highest souls, possessed reason or intellect, in addition to all of the lower principles of life. This last kind of soul was found only in human beings.

(Ferguson, 1993)

Aristotle viewed soul and body as form and matter; the soul was the organizing principle of the body. Soul and body could be distinguished in thought, not fact (because the soul cannot be observed and the body can be observed). For Plato the body is the instrument or vehicle of the soul: "I am soul: I have a body" (Robertson, 2009, p. 341). For Aristotle, there could not be body without soul or soul without body. This view had the advantage of preserving the human intact. Ferguson (1993) stated that this outlook created problems for Christian thought in the later Middle Ages. "Aristotle allowed that a part of the intellect might survive death, but his followers developed this in reference to the universal soul shared by individuals, and not as allowing an individual immortality" (Ferguson, 1993, p. 341).

Aristotle believed that the body existed before the soul but that the soul was superior. According to Kittel and Friedrich (1985), Aristotle felt that

> desire was good but should be restrained, for it was not the supreme good. The soul was a *soma* made up of the finest particles, and in *soma*, even apart from the soul, there was substance. Bodies were limited. The elements were bodies, and the universe was a body, with reason as it's soul.

### Stoics and Epicureans (334–263 BCE)

The two principle philosophical schools of the Hellenistic age were those of the Stoics and of the Epicureans. The Epicureans held that the soul was composed of atoms, just like everything else in the universe. But the atoms of the soul were thin and of various kinds: atoms of fire, air, breath, and very fine matter. The atoms were scattered throughout the body and controlled by a rational part that was located in the breast. In addition, all sensations of the body were the result of the soul. The soul was material and, therefore, could not be mortal. When the soul died and disintegrated, the soul atoms were scattered throughout the universe. Death was the end for both the body and the soul (Frost, 1962).

According to Frost (1962), the Stoics held that the human was both soul and body and that the soul was a spark from the divine fire controlled by a ruling part situated in the head. The soul of a human, the Stoics taught, was the source of what was known as perception, judgment, feeling, and will. The soul was rational and made the human able to think in terms of concepts and ideas. It made it possible for the human to make choices before acting. Frost (1962) further stated that Stoics held different ideas about immortality. Some thought that good and wise souls continued to exist after the death of the body, whereas other souls would perish with the body. Other Stoics believed that it did not matter if the soul was good or bad; they all lived until the end of the world.

### Plotinus (205–270 BCE)

Plotinus attempted to interpret the teachings of Plato. His work served as the foundation for a school known as *neo-Platoism*, or the new Platoism (Frost, 1962). Plotinus believed that the soul, wanting to be become a body occupied by a star, left its heavenly place and entered matter or a body. Frost (1962) said that from that state, the soul struggled to free itself from the body. When it succeeded, it returned to its star and dwelt there forever. If it failed, it descended lower and lower, moving from one body to another.

In summary, the philosophers mentioned in this section gave some insight into the belief about the earlier Greeks' thoughts about the relationship between the body and soul. The concept that there is a connection between the body and soul was a part of teachings of the great philosophers. They provided some earlier Christian influences into the holistic view of the body, mind, and soul (spirit) triad. One philosopher built ideas from the other, beginning with Homer. Homer taught that the soul was associated with breath; when the breath (soul) left the body, it made the body inactive (i.e., created death). The body was left behind at death when the soul was left to wander. Socrates believed that if a person did not receive a proper burial, the soul would simply wander aimlessly. Plato had the greatest influence on the early development of Christian thought because the doctrine of the immortality of the soul attracted Christians. Aristotle proposed that there could not be a body without a soul or a soul without a body. The two were very much a part of life. The Stoics and Epicureans thought that the soul of a human was the source of what was known as perception, judgment, feeling, and will. Finally, Plotinus believed that on death, the soul left the body, only to seek another. This introduced the concept of reincarnation.

## Theology of body and soul in the Bible

### *Body and the Old Testament*

The authors of the Old Testament spoke of human beings in terms of "flesh" and "soul." They used the word *gewiyya* (body) a few times, referring to the body of an angel (the word *flesh* would be inadequate) (Ezek. 1:11,23); to a slave in the sense of persons as manpower (Gen. 47:18); and to a corpse or carcass (Judg. 14:8,9). The Old Testament writers demonstrated little interest in distinguishing the body, as one part of a person, from the personality (*psyche*) as soul. To speak of a body made sense only to describe the person's capability as a worker at the disposal of a master or as a mere dead substance only to be buried. The body was just an object to be discarded after death.

The authors of the Old Testament believed that a person did not possess a soul and a body; rather, he or she was full of soul and flesh and replete with life and the potential activity but nevertheless threatened by illness and death. Freedman (1992) wrote that "soul without flesh is like a ghost without real existence, while flesh without soul is but a corpse" (p. 768). The authors of the Hebrew Bible were also not interested in the concept of the human being as an individual person, either as distinguished from other persons or as a small universe. Wherever a person was prominent in the Hebrew Bible, God elected that person. The idea of a person developing to a more perfect specimen of human being was foreign to the Hebrew Bible (Freedman, 1992).

Death was not understood as a separation of the divine soul from the mortal body. It remained a person's enemy, and only God was powerful: "My flesh and my heart may fail, but God is the rock of my heart and my portion forever" (Ps. 73:26).

The doctrine of creation set forth the essential corporeality of human existence. Adam and Eve were provided with physical bodies (Gen. 2:7, 22). The idea that God made physical bodies first and then breathed the breath of life into them meant that humans were living bodies and not incarnate souls. This doctrine put strong emphasis on the soul and on the idea that humankind was more than a living soul. The holistic relationship between body and soul undermined any thought that a human being was simply the sum of his or her parts.

Elwell (1996) stated that bodily existence not only is essential aspect of being human but also is God's perfect will. In the beginning, God pronounced that all creation was "very good" (Gen. 1:31). Therefore, to be truly human is to exist in bodily form. This divine affirmation of physical existence is opposed to any notion that the body is inferior to the spirit. According to Elwell (1996), unlike the views of the Gnostics of the 2nd and 3rd centuries CE[2] the Scriptures never represented the physical body as a prison from which the spirit must be freed. There was nothing inherently evil about the human body. Throughout the Old Testament, the body is presented as a gift from God (Ps. 139: 14–16).

Adam and Eve enjoyed a perfect fellowship with God, and that fellowship was experienced in the body (Gen. 1:27–31). The integration of body and soul constituted a remarkable internal dynamic that integrated the material and spiritual realms. The body became the expression of the soul (Elwell, 1996). The sin of Adam and Eve thus not only affected their spiritual status before God but had physical consequences as well. Death came, and the earth from which the body was formed was cursed (Gen. 2:17; 3:17–19). With regard to the final disposition of the body, the principle of "dust to dust" held true (Gen. 3:19).

### Soul and the Old Testament

In the Old Testament (Hebrew Bible),[3] the word *nepes* denoted breath; it was used 755 times. The word's root means "to breathe" in a physical sense. Breathing was seen as a decisive mark of a living creature; its cessation meant the end of life. Departure of breath was a metaphor for death. In the Greek Bible (a Greek translation of the Hebrew Bible), the two most common usages of *nepes* in the Old Testament were "soul" (428 times) and "life" (117 times) (Elwell, 1996). *Nepes* in the Hebrew Bible was never the "immortal soul" but simply the life principle of living beings. A mortal *was* a living soul, rather than *had* a soul. Hebrew thought saw a unified being and a profoundly complex being, a psychophysical being. This conceptualization can be observed in Genesis 1:20–21, in which the *living* (*nepes*) referred to animals and was translated as "living creatures." The same term was applied to creation of humankind in Genesis 2:7, in which dust was vitalized by the breath of God and made the dust a living being—a person (Kittel & Friedrich, 1985).

*Spirit* (Greek *ruah)* was used in the Hebrew Testament 389 times. It was used more often to refer to God (136 times) than to persons or animals (129 times). Its basic meaning was "wind" (113 times). For example, the word was used in

Genesis 3:8 when Adam and Eve walked in the garden at a breezy time of day, in Exodus 12:13 when an east wind brought locusts, and in Exodus 14:21 when a strong east wind divided the water of the Red Sea.

### Use of body in the New Testament

The New Testament leant toward the Greek usage of "body and soul" (*soma* and *psyche*), but it also used the more Hebraic phrases "flesh and spirit" (*sarx* and *pneuma*) or "body and spirit" (*soma* and *pneuma*). The term *pneuma* pointed to the spiritual dimension and the human potential to connect with the supernatural (God or a higher power). The New Testament addressed the unified being; *redemption* referred not to soul as abstracted from the body, but to the whole person. In many instances psyche indicated "life" or the human person rather than the "soul" (e.g., Matt. 6.25; Mark 3:4, 8:35–37). Hunter (1990) stated that immortality of the soul rests, like resurrection of the body, on God and that the New Testament implies a trichotomous humility compromising the body, soul, and spirit: the human being is a unified, although bipolar, being, and embodied life. First Thessalonians 5:23 supports Hunter's (1990) statement, "May the God of peace himself sanctify you entirely; and may your spirit and soul and body be kept sound and blameless at the coming of our Lord Jesus Christ." This seems to refer to the notion of the holistic health and welfare of the believer.

Elwell (1996) stated that the essential corporeality (i.e., tangible element) of human existence was set forth in the New Testament. In the Christian Bible, the incarnation[4] was God's ultimate endorsement of the physical body (Matt. 1:20–25; Luke 1:26–35; Rom. 1:3; Gal. 4:4; 1 Tim. 3:16; 1 John 4:2–3). Complete redemption meant the reclamation of humanness in the most comprehensive sense, and this mandated the "infleshing" of the Word (John 1:14). Jesus's body became the locus for God's redemptive activity in the world. It was both the temple and the sacrifice in that it manifested the glory of God and atoned for the sins of the world (Mark 12:22; Luke 22:19; John 1:14, 2:21; Rom. 3:24–25).

It appears that the term for the *body* was rarely used in Jesus's teaching (Freedman, 1992). There was, however, some emphasis on life in its bodily form—for example, Jesus's healing restored the body of a sick person (Mark 5:29), and the disciples' obedience involved their bodies (i.e., that they should not commit adultery [Matt. 5:29] or become the cause of anxiety [Matt. 6:25] or fear [Matt:10:28]). This idea was central to Paul's letters: to present one's body as a living sacrifice (but not in martyrdom). The body, not the soul, was the temple of the Holy Spirit (1 Cor. 6:19–20).

### Use of soul in the New Testament

The terms *soul* (Hebrew *nephesh* and Greek *psyche*) and *spirit* (Hebrew *ruach* and Greek *pneuma*) seem to have been used interchangeably at times in the New Testament (Bultmann, 1975). For example, in John 12:27, Jesus said, "Now is my soul troubled," whereas in the next chapter John said that Jesus was "troubled in spirit" (John 13:21). Similarly, Mary stated in Luke 1:46–47, "My soul magnifies the Lord, and my spirit rejoices in God my Savior." This seems to be an example of parallelism, in which the same idea is repeated with different but synonymous words (Grudem, 1994).

Jesus said not to fear those who "kill the body but cannot kill the soul" but to "fear him who can destroy both soul and body in hell" unless there were aspects of the person that lived on after the body was dead. Grudem (1994) stated that when Jesus talked about soul and body, he was referring to the entire person, even though he did not mention the spirit as a separate component. The word *soul* seemed to stand for the entire nonphysical part of the person.

God told the rich fool, "This night your soul is required of you" (Luke 12:20). Sometimes death was viewed as the returning of the spirit to God. So David could pray, in words later quoted by Jesus on the cross, "Into your hand I commit my spirit" (Luke 23:46). At death, "the spirit returns to God who gave it" (Eccl. 12:7). When Jesus was dying, "he bowed his head and gave up his spirit" (John 19:30), and likewise Stephen, before dying, prayed, "Lord Jesus, receive my spirit" (Acts 7:59).

A trichotomist might argue that these passages say different things. When a person died, both the spirit and soul did in fact go to heaven. Note, however, that nowhere did the scriptures say that the person's "soul and spirit" went to heaven or were yielded up by God.

If the soul and spirit were separate and distinct things, the reader would expect that such language would be affirmed somewhere in the Bible, if only to ensure that no essential part of the person would be left behind. Grudem (1994) stated that the Bible includes no such language and that the biblical writers (although, admittedly, it was edited by many various writers over time) did not seem to care whether the soul or the spirit departed at death, because both words seemed to mean the same thing.

## Theologians' view of body and soul

By the middle of the 2nd century, Christians were beginning to address the philosophical agenda of the soul. Christianity, as interpreted by the apologists (i.e., "defenders" of the faith), taught that the soul and body were separate and that the soul was a part of the person that most nearly represented the good in the universe. The soul was immortal but continued to live in a resurrected body. Death was not seen as a separation of the body and soul but as a purification of the body so that it might be a fit place for the soul to dwell throughout eternity (Frost, 1962).

The apologists were the first to make connections between Christianity and the Greek philosophers. For example, generally, an apologist explained the Christian reference to eating flesh and blood (i.e., that it did not mean cannibalism) and clarified that the talk of love did not mean wild orgies. The apologists had to make Christian theology seem intellectually respectable, and usually that meant relating it to Greek philosophy (Frost, 1962).

### Justin Martyr (died 165 CE)

Justin Martyr was an early apologist who observed the inconsistency between the Platonist doctrine of the eternity and incorruptibility of the soul and the Christian belief that the individual soul was generated, or had its beginning, in God's act of creation. Christianity maintained that if the soul survived death, it was only because God willed it to do so, not because of its intrinsic nature (Barnard, 1967; Placher, 1983). According to Martyr, the soul was a creation of God and did not originate from the stars or anything earthly.

### Origen (185–254 CE)

Origen believed that all souls achieved salvation, according to Plato's view that souls were the real self and that humans were born as new bodies again and again. Origen made history important. He saw the soul as a process by which God gave freedom to all creation and then guided humans to salvation without destroying that freedom. Origen believed that the soul was in its own natural incorporeal state; that the world that God created was a spiritual world consisting entirely of "rational beings"; and that the soul, united to earth in an earthly body, was just such a rational being (Ferguson, 1990). Moreover, Origen believed that the individual soul preexisted its embodiment. The soul was the seat of that which corresponds to the image of God. Philosophers influenced by Plato tended to regard the soul as the real human person, rather than as the union of soul and body. Origen departed from Plato by declining to acknowledge separate referents for the intellect and the soul.

### Augustine (354–430 CE)

In the West, Augustine of Hippo taught that the human was made of soul and body. The soul itself was the ultimate principle of life and of growth as well as the seat of the divine image. For Augustine, however, the body was a prison house of the soul and the source of all evil. The soul was immaterial (not made of matter), was wholly different and distinct from the body, and was "in no way inferior to the body" (Augustine, 1993, p. 82). Augustine repudiated the notion of corporeality of the soul and instead taught that the soul directed and formed the body (the doctrine of incorporeity); however, how this happened was a mystery (Frost, 1962).

Augustine also taught that each person had his or her own soul and that the soul was not an emanation from God. According to his belief, the soul did not exist before the body. Therefore preexistence of the soul was not an issue. Augustine believed that when the body was formed, the soul entered the body, and it lived there forever while it directed the body. He was drawn to the idea that each individual soul was directly created by God, but how the soul was created was a mystery to Augustine. The theologian was ambivalent about when the soul was created—whether at the time of its union with the body, ahead of time, or at the moment of creation itself. Ferguson (1990) found no evidence that Augustine ever resolved the issue of preexistence.

Augustine believed that the soul was immortal. In his book *On Free Choice of the Will*, he stated, "Both body and soul are formed by an unchangeable form that abides forever" (Augustine, 1993, p. 63). He taught that the life of the soul after the death of the body was either happy or miserable, depending on how the person had lived on earth. If, during this earthly existence, the person won the favor of God, he or she was given blessedness. If the person did not win the favor of God, he or she was condemned to misery (Frost, 1962). Augustine stated, "He [God] creates the souls that do not love him and perfects the souls that do love him" (Augustine, 1993, p. 109).

### *Thomas Aquinas (1225–1274 CE)*

Aquinas taught that the human soul was created by God. He believed that the soul was immaterial (not made of matter), part of the intellect, and a vital principle of the body. This intellectual soul was added to the body at birth. Although other souls exist, the human soul was different from all others in that it was intelligent and could will. Frost (1962) stated that this intelligent soul was not dependent on the body for its existence or functioning. This intellectual soul continued to act after the body ceased to exist. Moreover, the soul continued to exist just as it did while the body was alive. Thus, it formed a new body—a spiritual body that functioned through eternity. Catholicism accepted this view and made it fundamental to the church's teachings (Frost, 1962).

## Controversies regarding the soul

The 9th century saw controversies about the nature of the soul; one such controversy concerned incorporeity and the other individuality. Two parties in this theological debate were Ratramnus of Corbie and an anonymous writer from Reims, who might have been Archbishop Hincmar. At the request of a civil official, Ratramnus wrote a treatise declaring that the soul was incorporeal and was not circumscribed to the body. After reading Ratramnus's treatise, the official addressed some questions to a man from Reims (possibly Hincmar), who responded. The writer from Reims refuted the claims of Ratramnus and stated that the soul was tied to the body. This writer asserted that, through knowledge, the soul went beyond the boundaries of the body. That was the end of the debate; according to Gonzalez (1970), the only thing it demonstrated was that the Augustinian doctrine of incorporeity of the soul was in question again.

The problem of the individual soul was much more important, because the notion depended on the possibility of an individual, conscious life after death. Gonzalez (1970) recounted the argument between Ratramnus and an Irish monk named Marcius, who supported the theory of a universal soul, of which individual souls partook. The historical basis for the controversy was found in a text by Augustine that discussed the question of the number of souls and reached no clear conclusion. Debaters used this text to prove that the soul was at once one and multiple. By interpreting Augustine within the framework of neo-Platonic realism, they argued that there was a universal soul and that the individual soul only existed by participating in that universal soul.

The refutation of this argument was based not on Augustine's work but on Ratramnus's own position regarding universals (i.e., universal soul) and his interest in safeguarding human individuality. In keeping with Augustine, Ratramnus did not conceive of universals as real entities in the same sense in which particular things were real. The universal soul was one to which every living thing belonged—a collective. It composed both matter and form combined (Frost, 1962). When Augustine spoke of the soul in the singular, he did not refer to a universal soul that existed beyond particular souls "but referred to the concept of the soul—truly a concept, but not any more real than the individual souls, nor metaphysically prior to them" (Gonzalez, 1970, p. 125).

## Body and soul in the context of occupational therapy

The concept of body and spirit in occupational therapy has a biblical origin. The philosophy of treating the client holistically is therefore not a new concept in occupational therapy. The principle of treatment includes using techniques and theories from related research in the physical sciences to improve functioning in the clients' activities of daily living.

The therapist's theology about the relationship between the body and soul is very important. In the Hebrew Testament, the physical body was just matter to be discarded after death, because the soul had separated from it. The soul and body were seen as two separate entities that divided after the death of the body. If the therapist believes that the body and the soul are separate, and that the body is more important than the soul, he or she will feel that the physical needs of the soul are already met and will just treat the body, without regard to the client's spiritual needs. In the New Testament, however, the body and soul are a mutually interdependent unit. The two are united, not separated—one is as important and valued as the other. This is consistent with the concept of holism and what makes a living person soulful. Therefore, the therapist must treat the person holistically by including the spiritual dimension. I believe that spirituality is an occupation, not a performance component, as suggested by the Canadian Association of Occupational Therapists. How the spiritual dimension is included in the treatment of clients is a matter of the theology of occupation.

## Summary

This chapter began by identifying terms used to describe the body and soul used in various sacred texts. The Christian Bible, the Koran, and the sacred texts of the Hindu and Buddhist traditions address the relationship between body and soul. The religious traditions that address the relationship between the body and soul also include the concept of holism in their beliefs about health. It was the

Greek philosophers who proposed the concept of the soul, and it was the Christian apologists who related the Greek philosophy to the beliefs of Christian theology. The debates about when the soul enters the body—at conception or at birth—continues today.

The relationship between the body and soul is not about a belief that the body has no use and can be disregarded, but about an integral and interactive relationship. It has implications for beliefs about health policy, including social issues such as abortion, birth control, euthanasia, right to suicide, reproductive practices, surrogate mothers, transplants, and involuntary mental hospitalization. These and other health issues can affect the course of therapy in many practice areas. Culture and its relation to health and religious practices are discussed in greater detail in Chapter 7.

Beliefs about holism also involve one's attitudes, worldview, and religious tradition. It seems that holism—the mind, body and spirit (soul)—is universal among clients who have a religious tradition; at the same time, a client does not have to have a religious tradition to believe in a relationship between the mind, body, and spirit (soul). The therapist must inquire about the client's holistic perspective during the evaluation process. As suggested in Chapter 1, it can be assumed that the client is on a spiritual journey, and spiritual health practices should be identified. The soul (spirit) is as important in occupational therapy as the body, and one can view the spirit (soul) as an occupation.

## Notes

1 Pythagoras and his followers (known as Orphics) were early Greek philosophers who believed that the destiny of the soul after leaving the body was determined by the life in the body. They had rules that were to be followed that ensured desirable existence after death (Frost, 1962).
2 Gnoticism was a movement during the early church period featuring views that were focused on the quest for secret knowledge transmitted only to the "enlighted" and marked by the view that matter is evil. Gnostics denied the humanity of Jesus (McKim 1996).
3 "Hebrew Bible" is a term for the canonical writing that Christians refer to as the Old Testament. The Jewish canon of Hebrew Scriptures has 24 books divided among Torah (5), Prophets (8), and Writings (11), which appear in modern translation as 39 books (McKim, 1996).
4 The doctrine that the eternal second Person of the Trinity became a human being and "assumed flesh" in Jesus of Nazareth. The doctrine holds that Jesus was one divine person with both a divine and a human nature (McKim, 1996).

## References

Augustine. (1993). *On free choice of the will* (T. Williams, Trans.). Indianapolis, IN: Hackett.
Barnard, L. W. (1967). *Justin Martyr: His life and thought.* London: Cambridge University Press.
Bultmann, R. (1975). *History and eschatology: The presence of Eternity (1954–1955) (Gifford lectures).* New York: Harper Greenwood.

Cullmann, O. (1958). *Immortality of the soul.* New York: Macmillan.

Elwell, W. (Ed.). (1996). *Baker theological dictionary of the Bible.* Grand Rapids, MI: Baker.

Ferguson, E. (Ed.). (1990). *Encyclopedia of early Christianity.* New York: Garland.

Ferguson, E. (1993). *Backgrounds of early Christianity.* Grand Rapids, MI: William B. Eerdmans.

Freedman, D. (1992). *The Anchor Bible dictionary* (Vol. 5). New York: Doubleday.

Frost, S. (1962). *Basic teachings of the great philosophers.* New York: Doubleday.

Gonzalez, J. (1970). *A history of Christian thought: From the beginnings to the Council of Chalcedon.* Nashville, TN: Abingdon Press.

Grudem, W. (1994). *Systematic theology: An introduction to biblical doctrine.* Grand Rapids, MI: Zondervan.

Homer. (1984). *The Iliad* (D. B. Hull, Trans.). Scottsdale, AZ: D. B. Hull. (Original work 800 BC.)

Hunter, R. (Ed.). (1990). *Dictionary of pastoral care and counseling.* Nashville, TN: Abingdon Press.

Kittel, G., & Friedrich, G. (1985). *Theology dictionary of the New Testament.* Grand Rapids, MI: William B. Eerdmans.

McKim, D. K. (1996). *Westminster dictionary of theological terms.* Louisville, KY: Westminster John Knox Press.

Musser, D., & Price, J. (Eds.). (1992). *A new handbook of Christian theology.* Nashville, TN: Abingdon Press.

Pagels, E. (1997). *The Gnostic gospels.* New York: Vintage Books.

Placher, W. (1983). *A history of Christian theology.* Philadelphia: Westminster Press.

Plato. (1977). *Timaeus and Critias* (D. Lee, Trans.). New York: Penguin Books.

Robertson, D. (2009). Plato on conversation and experience. *Philosophy, 84*(3), 355–369.

Schimmel, A. (1975). *Mystical dimensions of Islam.* Chapel Hill: University of North Carolina Press.

Smith, H. (1991). *The world's religion.* San Francisco: HarperCollins.

Tillich, P. (1968). *A history of Christian thought: From its Judaic and Hellenistic origins to existentialism.* New York: Simon & Schuster.

# 4 Therapeutic self

At the 1956 Allenberry Workshop Conference in Boiling Springs, Pennsylvania, entitled "The Function and Preparation of the Psychiatric Occupational Therapist," an entire session was devoted to the use of the self as a therapeutic tool. The Preparatory Commission's report on the use of self noted,

> The therapist's personality is the most important tool in any therapeutic setting. While the use of activities is a differentiating mark of the occupational therapist, activities are effective only to the extent that the occupational therapist as an active participant in the treatment situation is able to bring to it a genuine warmth, understanding, flexibility and objectivity. Implicit in a satisfactory therapeutic relationship between therapist and patient is the therapist's awareness and understanding of himself as a human being, with recognition and understanding of his needs and feelings in interpersonal relationships... Since the OT's feelings are an important factor, treatment formulations cannot be rigid. He must be comfortable in whatever techniques he uses, be able to recognize his limitations, to accept and work within them if they or the situation cannot or should not be changed.
>
> (West, 1959, p. 27)

The report seems to suggest that the therapist's training or particular school or theory of therapy does not make a difference; rather, the ability to be "human" is of prime importance to success in treatment. The studies of Carkhuff and Truax (1967) agree with this assumption. Looking at various therapeutic orientations, Dreyfus (1967) wrote that all of them failed to demonstrate their own efficacy and explained that a single variable—humanness—seemed to underlie all therapeutic approaches and could account for the positive result obtained by all.

In the clinical setting, the relationship between the client and clinician can be viewed as a relationship between souls. The spiritual self is the manifestation of the soul of each person; the soul is the divine self. Therefore, the therapeutic encounter invites a reciprocal relationship between two souls. Occupations become meaningful when they encounter the soul. When an occupation becomes meaningful, it is sustained and will be repeated. Occupations are then expressed as the spiritual self in the outer world. Therefore, the soul expresses itself in the spiritual self through occupation (see Figure 4.1). This is accomplished through the therapeutic use of self. *Use of self* refers to the various interpersonal dynamics between therapist and client and the impact and use of these dynamics in intervention (Swarbrick & Burkhardt, 2000). The therapist's use of self is critical to engaging the client in occupation.

Three ingredients are essential to establishing a therapeutic relationship: neutrality, empathy, and caring (Siegel, 1988). As Siegel (1988) explained these principles, the therapist accepts the client; is tolerant of and interested in the client's painful emotions; and, finally, is able, through reflection, to communicate to the client what the client expects from the therapist. By remaining neutral but engaged, the therapist encourages the client to interact (Siegel, 1988). The therapeutic use of self is more than just a relationship based on mutual respect. It is intentional and uses the self to recognize the higher self in the therapist and the client.

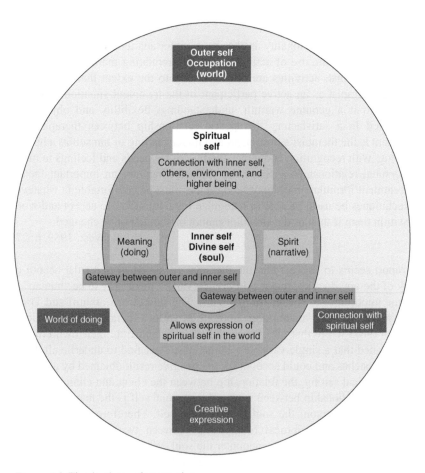

*Figure 4.1* The theology of occupation.

The therapeutic relationship, then, can be described as recognizing a client's true self (soul) by understanding his or her spiritual self. McColl (2003) stated that if spirituality were not about the essence of the true self (inner world soul) but about the ability to transcend the spiritual self (outer world), then it would be about the recognition of a power greater than the spiritual self. The therapist would perceive the true self in relation to the outer world.

The therapeutic use of self is the "glue" that holds the relationship among the therapist, the client, and a transcendent being (soul) together in the therapeutic relationship. In describing this triadic relationship, Fowler (1981) stated that human communities have a faith structure that is triangular in nature. In communities, the soul is connected to others by shared trust and loyalty. Both the soul and others (i.e., people) are mediated, strengthened, and realized by the shared trust in and loyalty to a higher power. The triangle between the therapist, client, and soul takes place in a community; is accessed through occupation; and is made possible by the therapeutic use of self. The community is the therapeutic environment. It can be the patient's home, work, or clinic. The therapist enters the environment where the patient's spirituality takes place. The therapist taps into the patient's spirituality where occupations are used. The therapeutic use of self holds the relationship together during the treatment process through occupations. Intentionality (the self) operationalizes the spirituality between the client and therapist. *Intentionality* means the conscious application of the will or intent to direct the self to engage the self/soul of the "other."

According to Punwar and Peloquin (2000), "to know the self, to cultivate the best of one's abilities in order to help, is an important part of therapy" (p. 42). Knowing the self means that the therapist becomes aware of his or her spiritual development and its impact on the client during therapy. Developing and becoming aware of one's own spiritual path will help therapists integrate spirituality into the treatment process and, in so doing, perhaps enhance the outcome. Understanding one's own spiritual development is an important part of being a therapist: "The conscious use of self involves planning one's personal responses so as to help a patient" (Mosey, 1986, p. 42).

The therapist is like any other tool used in treatment. Although the client–therapist relationship is not ordinarily considered the central focus of treatment, it is a primary and necessary ingredient in the therapeutic process. Spector (1996) stated that "without a successful relationship, change in a patient's condition is unlikely to occur" (p. 21).

The therapist's personality is the most important tool in the treatment setting. The therapeutic use of self is important enough to be mentioned in the *Occupational Therapy Practice Framework: Domain and Process* (American Occupational Therapy Association, 2002, 2008, 2014). To use the therapeutic self, therapists must be on their own personal faith journey in that they must be aware of themselves as spiritual beings and be able to recognize their own spirituality in the therapeutic relationship. Through the therapeutic self, the therapist and client can access the self, and spiritual growth can occur. The self in each individual is a reciprocal relationship. An example would be when a therapist uses an occupation that becomes spiritual to the client and that client realizes that the occupation is essential to his or her spiritual well-being. It can be as simple as taking care of a pet, gardening, a sport activity, or bird watching.

West (1959, p. 1) listed the following requirements or conditions needed for the effective use of self:

- Self-understanding, including abilities and limitations; awareness of one's own needs; and ability to meet these satisfactorily
- Warmth, flexibility in relationships (give and take), basic personality security
- Knowledge of personality development
- Acceptance of the client as a person
- Dedication of humility
- A constant eagerness to search for knowledge
- A particular skill, in which one is thoroughly comfortable, so that one can provide a sense of security in the use of all skills and offer a basis for relating to the client.

As the therapist matures, he or she uses his or her attitude more effectively, uses the self in a more developed manner, and becomes more comfortable being in a relationship with the client. The therapist develops a sense of responsibility for increasing his or her understanding in the area of practice. Occupations are essential for the use of self to be effective and the client's spirituality to be expressed. Moreover, the effective use of the self is determined or limited by the therapist's theology as well as his or her knowledge and skill in recognizing his or her own spiritual path. Effective use can also be determined or limited by the physical setting, environmental milieu, relationship among disciplines, and ability to express oneself effectively. Devereaux (1989, p. 196) gave the elements of therapeutic relationships as follows:

- Competence—being competent in the field in which one is practicing is a part of caring. It nourishes our clients and ourselves;
- Belief in the dignity and worth of the individual—honoring the client's integrity and realizing his or her need for mastery and control;
- Belief that each person has the potential for change and growth—provide the means for the client to adapt through occupation toward health and wellness;
- Communication—listen to the client in a way that identifies cultural and health practices;
- Values—understand the client's religious beliefs, for they reflect how he or she lives and provide the standard for living and meaning for occupation;
- Touch—recognize that touch is a powerful tool but must be used with caution;
- Sense of humor—do not take oneself seriously. Add humor to lessen the tension and fear during the treatment session.

The relationship in the therapeutic environment is the core of human needs. Despite occupational therapy's history of emphasizing caring relationships, its focus has been on health care delivery defined by the biomedical model, illness curing, and finances. Recognizing the need to move away from the business and medical model, two groups, the Fetzer Institute and the Pew Health Professions Commission, formed a task force to develop a new health paradigm. One result of this collaboration was the concept of relationship-centered care (RCC). According to Manning-Walsh et al. (2004), "RCC is healthcare in which relationships are valued and attended to and includes relationships between and among practitioners, patients, and their families" (p. 26). RCC suggests that caring is a manifestation of being in the world. Caring focuses attention on the mind, body, and spirit and "includes being as well as knowing and doing" (Roach, 1998, p. 30; Watson, 1999, p. 455). Moreover, "caring is understood as value-laden relations of infinite responsibility to self and others" (Watson & Smith, 2002, p. 455) and is an essential human attribute and a total way of being (Roach, 1998). RCC moves caring one step further and emphasizes the importance of relating and "interactions among people as foundational to therapeutic or healing activities" (Manning-Walsh et al., 2004, p. 27).

The main principles of RCC are respect, awareness, and understanding of self, with particular attention to the caring of self. RCC entails a commitment to personal growth and development—a commitment to nourishing the mind, body, and spirit so the person can establish relationships with others in a soulful manner. It requires a conscious effort to understand the self, to understand the personal spiritual journey, and to engage in self-analysis. When a person can understand and value the self, he or she has a deeper appreciation in relationship to others. A soulful person can then interact with the soulfulness of another person. When there is a connection between each soul, the therapist can begin to learn from the client, and reciprocal learning takes place. An RCC therapist learns from the other person and so becomes a student of the other. The therapist and client become teacher and learner to each other. Therapists can form such a relationship with their client, with another professional, or with the community. The client's story about his or her illness experience becomes more important in reciprocal learning because it adds meaning to health. When the client becomes the teacher and expert, the therapist listens and hears the client's story. In the context of this story, the therapist learns about the client's illness experiences, meaning in life, religious traditions, and worldview.

When reciprocal learning occurs, a higher level of relationship is achieved, and *mutuality*, defined as "having the same relationship each to the other, a relationship that is reciprocal" (Manning-Walsh et al., 2004, p. 28), is found. Mutuality allows for the establishment of goals for the good of the therapist and client. It includes a shared commonality and acceptance of differences in spiritual traditions. The client's and therapist's values, culture, customs, and religious traditions are shared and respected, and vice versa.

Palmer (2004) suggested that the therapist must strip away the ego so that he or she is interacting with the client at the soulful level. To do this, the therapist needs to be reminded of the following seven rules, which were inspired from attending numerous seminars:

1   Never ask a question when one knows the answer.
2   Never give advice or even ask a question that implies giving advice.
3   Do not ask questions out of curiosity.
4   Never ask a question for the purpose of making a point, such as questions that begin with "have you considered … ?"
5   Be brief and to the point.
6   Remember that the client's nonverbal behaviors are irrelevant and can easily lead the client down a false path.
7   Refrain from problem solving.

These rules prevent the therapist from doing or saying anything that draws attention away from the client.

At the heart of the RCC model is the self. The RCC model is different from the patient-centered model, in which the client is the focus of the relationship. The RCC model understands the self in the context of the person's culture, family, ethnicity, gender, beliefs, values, and religious tradition. Self-care is paramount to the RCC concept. Orem (1991) defined self-care as "a process that includes activities that individuals personally initiate and perform on their own behalf in maintaining life, health, and well-being" (p. 365). Self-care activities help the therapist self-assess, become self-aware, and develop a personal worldview. Through this process, the therapist can become aware of his or her own spiritual development and its impact on the client during therapy.

## Summary

This chapter discusses the role of the therapeutic use of self. The use of self has been a part of the history of occupational therapy and remains a vital element of the therapeutic process. The RCC model is different from the patient-centered model in that the focus is the self. With a healthy self, the therapist is better able to develop a therapeutic relationship with the client. In addition, the therapist's soulful self interacts with the soulful self of others, including clients, other professionals, and the community.

The concept of relationship-centered care will be used throughout the book instead of client-centered care. Relationship-centered care is more consistent with current thought and emphasizes the importance of the therapist's self-care. The relationship-centered model emphasizes the need to care for the self in order to care for others.

The next chapter examines spiritual development and its relationship to the self. Spiritual development is an integral part of learning how to know the self and how to take care of the self so that the therapeutic self can be used in the clinical setting.

# References

American Occupational Therapy Association. (2002). Occupational therapy practice framework: Domain and process. *American Journal of Occupational Therapy, 56,* 609–639.

American Occupational Therapy Association. (2008). Occupational therapy practice framework: Domain and process (2nd ed.). *American Journal of Occupational Therapy, 62,* 625–683.

American Occupational Therapy Association. (2014) Occupational therapy practice framework: Domain and process (3rd ed.). *American Journal of Occupational Therapy, 68,* s12.

Carkhuff, R., & Truax, C. (1967). *Toward effective counseling and psychotherapy: Training and practices.* Chicago: Aldin.

Devereaux, E. (1989). Occupational therapy's challenge: The caring relationship. *American Journal of Occupational Therapy, 38,* 791–798.

Dreyfus, E. (1967). Humanness: A therapeutic variable. *Personnel and Guidance Journal, 45,* 573–578.

Fowler, J. (1981). *Stages of faith: The psychology of human development and the quest for meaning.* San Francisco: Harper.

McColl, M. (2003). Spirit, occupation, and disability. In R. P. Pleming Cottrell (Eds.), *Perspectives for occupation-based practice* (pp. 243–253). Bethesda, MD: AOTA Press.

Manning-Walsh, J., Wagenfeld-Heintz, E., Asmus, A., Chambers, M., Reed, W., & Wylie, J. (2004). Relationship-centered care: The expanding cup model. *International Journal for Human Caring, 8*(2), 26–31.

Mosey, A. (1986). *Psychosocial components of occupational therapy.* New York: Raven Press.

Orem, D. (1991). *Nursing concepts of practice* (3rd ed.). New York: McGraw-Hill.

Palmer, P. (2004). *The hidden wholeness.* San Francisco: Jossey-Bass.

Punwar, A., & Peloquin, S. (2000). *Occupational therapy principles and practice* (3rd ed.). New York: Lippincott Williams & Wilkins.

Roach, M. (1998). Caring ontology: Ethics and the call of suffering. *International Journal for Human Caring, 2*(2), 30–34.

Siegel, B. (1988). *Love, medicine and miracles: Lessons learned about self-healing from a surgeon's experience with exceptional patients.* New York: Harper & Row.

Spector, M. (1996). Developing therapeutic use of self through spirituality. *Journal of Occupational Therapy Students,* 21–26.

Swarbrick, P., & Burkhardt, A. (2000). Spiritual health: Implications for the occupational therapy process. *Mental Health Special Interest Section Quarterly, 23*(2), 1–3.

Watson, J. (1999). *Postmodern nursing and beyond.* London: Churchill Livingstone.

Watson, J., & Smith, M. (2002). Caring science and the science of unitary human beings: A trans-theoretical discourse for nursing knowledge development. *Journal of Advanced Nursing, 37,* 452–461.

West, W. (1959). Use of self as a therapeutic tool. In W. West (Ed.), *Changing concepts and practice in psychiatric occupational therapy* (pp. 26–37). Dubuque, IA: William C. Brown.

# 5 Theories of spiritual development

## Chapter objectives

1 Explain four theories of spiritual development (Moody & Carroll, Assagioli, Peck, Fowler).
2 Apply the four theories of spiritual development to health care and health care practice and practitioner interaction with the client in context.

In occupational therapy practice, it is important to recognize clients' level of spiritual and faith development. Knowing about faith development is consistent with the concept of occupational science, because the development of faith can be observed. Faith is an activity and can involve objects such as prayer beads, amulets, and songbooks. This chapter reviews the views on spiritual development of Moody and Carroll (1997), Assagioli (1973, 1976), Peck (1987, 1997), and Fowler (1981). These thinkers serve as the most comprehensive examples, and they each held different views about spiritual development.

## Moody and Carroll's theory of spiritual development

Since civilization began, humans have recognized a structure to the life course from infancy though old age. The idea of life stages has long been expressed through symbols, myths, and rituals, whereas modern societies rely on the social sciences as well as culture to suggest a way of life. Moody and Carroll (1997) stated that people develop a way of life according to how they conceive the role of purpose and meaning in life. This search for meaning must be recognized as the driving force in the construction of new paradigms for growth and development over the life course. The urge to find a deeper purpose in life unfolds in a sequence of stages that exerts a slow but sure metamorphic effect on the adult personality. In the end, one who passes through these stages emerges more fulfilled and self-realized (Moody & Carroll, 1997).

Carl Jung (1933/1957) was the first psychotherapist to seriously attempt to describe a spiritual sequence in the life course. Jung pointed out that the spiritual process begins in people almost automatically. When youthful illusions are shed and repressed, childhood ideals resurface, and meanings in life are reexamined.

Early interests and ambitions lose their fascination, and mature ones take their place. A person gropes toward wisdom and begins a search for enduring personal values.

According to Moody and Carroll (1997), spiritual development is characterized by five stages: (1) the call, (2) the search, (3) the struggle, (4) the breakthrough, and (5) the return. The call is known by many names—conversion, summons, and change of heart. The search is a quest for a spiritual practice that seems right. It takes place on a deeper level, so that one is looking for something that one cannot easily put in words but senses it out there somewhere, someplace, waiting, calling. The struggle is the way (method). Seekers who are on a quest are tested, endure trials, and are challenged. The breakthrough comes when the spiritual forces collecting inside the seeker can no longer be held in check. A sudden surge of energy pushes things to the limit; then follows a burst of vision, and the hidden forces become more conscious. Something has changed, and the person is not the same. The return from this quest occurs to the ordinary, everyday life goes on as before, yet with a different level of understanding and perception. In the context of occupational therapy, the return is found in participation in the activities of daily life. The person's occupations take on a silent language of the ordinary in the way he or she dresses, eats a meal, engages in a leisure activity, or participates in a religious activity.

## Assagioli's theory of spirituality over the life course

Another psychotherapist, Roberto Assagioli (1973, 1976), made spirituality in the life course a dominant part of his therapeutic method. Like Jung (1933/1957), Assagioli (1973, 1976) believed that the search for life's purpose could only begin only after a person had lived long enough and made enough mistakes to recognize that an unexamined life goes nowhere. The change often begins with a growing sense of dissatisfaction, a feeling that something is missing. This missing piece is nothing material or definite; it is something vague and elusive that the person is unable to describe. Eventually, this disquieting inner pressure sends the person on a search for the soul. Assagioli (1973, 1976) believed that this search only occurs between ages 30 and 40.

## Peck's theory of spiritual growth

Scott Peck (1987, 1997) described four stages of spiritual growth: (1) chaotic and antisocial; (2) formal and institutional; (3) skeptic and individual; and (4) mystic and communal. The chaotic stage is a primitive stage, in which people seem to be either religious or secular. Their belief system is superficial, and they are essentially unprincipled. Most young children and one in five adults fall into this stage (Peck, 1987). The chaotic stage is a time of undeveloped spirituality; Peck called it antisocial because adults in this stage seem generally incapable of loving others. They may appear loving and think of themselves that way, but their relationships with their fellow humans are all essentially manipulative and self-serving. This stage is chaotic because people in this stage are unprincipled and lack integrity.

Stage 2 is a stage of the letter of the law, in which religious fundamentalists are to be found. Conversion is often sudden, dramatic, and the process seems to be unconscious. If it is conscious, the person is in pain and prefers anything to the chaos of Stage 1. According to Peck (1987, 1997), most churchgoers are believers in Stage 2. They are attached to forms of religion, which is why Peck (1987, 1997) called this stage formal and institutional. They are so attached to canons and liturgy that they become upset if changes are made in the words, the music, or the traditional order of things.

Another characteristic of the religious behavior of people in the second stage is that their vision of God is almost entirely that of an external, transcendent being. They have little understanding of an immanent, indwelling God—God of the Holy Spirit, or what the Quakers call the Inner Light. Although they consider God loving, they also generally feel that God possesses—and will use—punitive power. This is precisely the kind of God they need—just as they need a legalistic religion for their governance. The principles of their parents' religion are figuratively engraved on their hearts—what psychotherapists call *internalized.* People of any faith can be at the second stage.

Once religion is internalized, usually around late adolescence, people become self-governing. They no longer depend on an institution for their governance. They begin to ask questions such as, "Who needs this church and its silly superstitions?" They then convert to Stage 3 or become atheists or agnostics.

People in Stage 3—skeptic, individual—are often scientifically minded, rational, moral, and humane. Their outlook is predominantly materialistic. They tend not only to be skeptical of the spiritual but uninterested in anything that cannot be proven. People in Stage 3 are often deeply involved in and committed to social causes. They make up their own mind and do not believe everything they read or hear. As advanced Stage 3 people, they are truth seekers. When they are able to find what they are seeking, they begin conversion to Stage 4.

Stage 4, the mystic communal stage, is the most mature stage. In this phase, people begin to doubt their own doubts. They feel connected to an unseen order of things, although they cannot fully define it. People at this stage are comfortable with the mystery of the sacred. They perceive that a unity underlies connectedness between things; between men and women, between people and other creatures, and even between people and inanimate matter. They acknowledge the enormity of the unknown and are not afraid of it, but they seek further understanding. They love mystery and will enter into religion to approach mystery. They are aware that the whole world is a community and realize that what divides humans into warring camps is precisely the lack of this awareness.

Peck (1987, 1997) stressed that people retain in themselves vestiges of the previous stages through which they have come. To acknowledge this existence is to integrate what Jung (1933/1957) called the "shadow." A person's development through these spiritual or religious stages is called *conversion.* During the conversion from Stage 3 to Stage 4, people generally first become conscious that such a thing as spiritual growth exists and that they can direct the process themselves. Conversions have one thing in common: a sense on the part of the person converted that their own conversions were not something they achieved themselves but were rather gifts from God.

## Fowler's theory of faith development

The last theory relevant to spiritual development is that of Fowler's (1981) faith stages. Fowler (1981) defined faith as

> the process of constitutive–knowing underlying a person's composition and maintenance of a comprehensive frame (or frames) of meaning generated from the person's attachments or commitments to centers of supra-ordinate value which have power to unify his or her experiences, thereby endowing the relationships, contexts, and patterns of everyday life, past and future, with significance.
>
> (pp. 25–26)

Fowler is saying that faith is relational and involves experiences with diverse people, institutions (church), events in people's lives, and everyday experiences. Faith is a way of discerning and committing to values that order the forces in people's lives. Fowler (1981) states, "Faith forms a way of seeing our everyday life in relation to holistic images of what we may call the ultimate environment" (p. 24)

Fowler (1981, p. xiii) was clear that faith development occurs in a primary group, in a particular culture, and through responses to initiatives of spirit and grace that are transcendent. Faith is not necessarily a religious phenomenon, but it is an imaginative reality that enables a person to see "him- or herself in relation to others against a background of shared meaning and purpose" (Fowler, 1981, p. 4). By *faith*, Fowler (1981) did not mean dogma or a particular theology or ideology. Faith is viewed as triadic and is a person's fundamental orientation to the environment, to the self, and to other people. It involves style of being, mode of valuing, and patterns of loyalty.

Fowler (1981) distinguished between belief and faith. *Belief* is a holding of ideas. Belief in a religious context comes out of the effort to translate experiences of the relation to transcendence into concepts and propositions. Fowler (1981) stated that "belief may be one of the ways faith expresses itself. *Faith* is the relation of trust in and loyalty to the transcendent about which concepts or propositions—beliefs—are fashioned" (p. 11).

Faith is more comprehensive and holistic than belief or religion. An Islamic, Jewish, Buddhist, or Christian religious affiliation manifests itself more in distinctions among life orientation, trust, fear, creativity, and nihilism than in creedal affirmation. As Fowler (1981) noted, "faith is an orientation of the total person, giving purpose and goal to one's hopes and strivings, thoughts and actions" (p. 14).

Fowler (1981) discussed faith as a human phenomenon, an apparently generic consequence of the universal human burden of finding or making meaning. He called attention to faith as being everywhere and being a relational matter. He believed that the patterns of faith that make selfhood possible and sustain identities are conventional (triadic) in form. Finally, faith is imagination, because it encompasses a felt image of an ultimate environment (community; Fowler, 1981, p. 33). There is a relationship between the self, the environment (or other beings), and a transcendent being. It is a reciprocal relationship and is ever-changing.

Fowler's (1981) faith stages look across the lifespan. Faith development is an ongoing process of "forming and reforming ... ways of being in and seeing the world" (p. 37). Beyond infancy and undifferentiated faith, Fowler (1981) described six stages of faith development:

1   Intuitive—projective faith
2   Mythic—literal faith
3   Synthetic—conventional faith
4   Individual—reflective faith
5   Conjunctive faith
6   Universalizing faith.

Fowler (1981) used the theories of Piaget (1976), Kohlberg (1968), and Erikson (1963) to explain each stage.

Stage 1, intuitive-projecting faith, is typical of a child 3 to 7 years old. This phase is fantasy filled, episodic, and highly imitative. The child in this stage is influenced by the attitudes, actions, gestures, values, and love of significant others in the primary environment. The transition to Stage 2 is the emergence of operational thinking. At the heart of the transition is the distinction between what is real and what only seems to be.

Stage 2, mythic-literal faith, usually happens by age 10, but the timing can vary. The child constructs a world in which order and disorder, good and evil, reward and punishment are explicit and literal—a world of dichotomies. Episodes acquire a linear continuity in a structure of meaning that persists. An elemental sense of fairness and justice that is based on the reciprocity emerges. According to Fowler (1981), "the new capacity or strength in this stage is the rise of narrative and the emergence of story, drama, and myth as ways of finding and giving coherence to experience" (p. 149).

The transition to Stage 3 is characterized by the emergence of formal operational thought, which makes reflection possible. Fowler (1981) noted that: the emergence of mutual interpersonal perspective taking ("I see you seeing me; I see me as you see me; I see you seeing me as you see me; I see you seeing me seeing you") creates the need for a more personal relationship with the unifying power of the ultimate environment (p. 150).

Stage 3, synthetic-conventional faith, is the "identity crisis," as Erikson (1963) called it. It occurs in relation to puberty, and the teenage years. The adolescent's religion involves a God who knows, accepts, and confirms the self deeply and who serves as an infinite guarantor of the self, with its forming myth of personal identity and faith. In other words, authorities outside the self provide the values and norms that one accepts without question. Fowler, (1981) wrote that:

> when God is a significant other in this mix—and the divine is always potentially what James Cone has called the "Decisive Other"—the commitment to God and the correlated self-image can exert a powerful ordering on a youth's identity and values outlook.
>
> (p. 154)

Symbols of country, social group, race, or religion have meaning and contribute to the identity of self. A system of informing images and values through which teens are committed remains principally a tacit system. *Tacit knowing* is a part of knowing that guides and shapes choices but of which one can give no account. That is, a person cannot tell how he or she knows through tacit knowing. Fowler (1981) stated that much of the church and synagogue life is included in Stage 3.

The transition to Stage 4 is a result of serious clashes or contradictions between valued authority sources and is marked by changes of leaders, policies, or practices previously deemed sacred. Growth is brought about by "the encounter with experiences or perspectives that lead to critical reflection on how one's beliefs and values have formed and changed, and on how 'relative' they are to one's particular group or background" (Fowler, 1981, p. 164).

In Stage 4 (individual-reflective faith), tacit values and meaning begin to be replaced by an explicit system. This stage marks the age of adulthood, although the actual age in years is irrelevant because some people never reach this stage. For a genuine move to occur, the person's reliance on external sources of authority must be interrupted. Instead, authority is relocated to within the self. The person forms a kind of internal "panel of experts"—called an *executive ego*—who reserve the right to choose and take responsibility for the person's choices. People in this stage retain the mutual interpersonal perspective from Stage 3, but they add awareness that the self has an ideology or worldview that has formed and re-formed over time. Stage 4 also adds an understanding of social relations in system terms. A person is Stage 4 thinks in terms of impersonal imperatives of laws, rules, and standards that govern social roles. The person engages in critical questioning and reflection, asking about symbols, "But what does it mean?" Fowler (1981) wrote that "if the symbol or symbolic act is truly meaningful, Stage 4 believes its meanings can be translated into propositions, definitions, and/or conceptual foundations" (p. 180). Through individual critical reflection, a strong self-worth is augmented by a strong sense of self-determination. Fowler (1981) stated that this transition, if it occurs, takes place in the person's 30s or 40s.

People in transition between Stages 3 and 4 find themselves with anarchic and disturbing inner voices. Stories, symbols, myths, and paradoxes from their own tradition or others' traditions challenge their previous faith development. They are disillusioned with the compromises they have made and recognize that life is more complex than they previously thought. They now take a dialectical and multilevel approach to life.

Fowler (1981) cited Chirban (1980), who showed that the further one moves beyond this stage, the more likely one is to exhibit an increased commitment to faith. Using the distinction between intrinsic and extrinsic forms of religious motivation, Chirban found that at Stage 4 and beyond, the incidence of extrinsic motivation virtually disappears. Intrinsic motivation (loyalty and commitment to one's worldview as true, regardless of whether it brings benefits or blame) characterizes post-conventional faith (Fowler, 1981, p. 300).

Stage 5, conjunctive faith, as a way of seeing, of knowing, of committing, moves beyond the dichotomizing logic of Stage 4's "either or" knowing. It sees both sides of an issue simultaneously ... suspects that things are organically related to each other; it attends to the pattern of interconnectedness in things (Fowler, 1981, p. 185).

This stage usually happens before a person is in midlife but can occur during midlife. Fowler (1981) said that he found Stage 5 difficult to describe. The egocentric self-confidence of Stage 4 is replaced by receptivity and trust in communal and dialogical relations. People in Stage 5 make their experience of truth the principle by which they test other claims to truth. They reclaim and rework their past and open themselves to the voices of their "deeper self" (Fowler, 1981, p. 198). People in this stage reintegrate the self to a wider awareness of people and issues and have considerably less aggressiveness in their life stance. They are able to affirm others in spite of disagreements.

Fowler (1981) stated that Stage 6, universalizing faith, is exceedingly rare. People in Stage 6 are drawn by God to universal love and justice, to the point of being heedless of self-preservation. People at this level not only reach a universalizing faith for themselves but make it available to others. Fowler (1981, p. 201) mentioned Mahatma Gandhi, Martin Luther King Jr., Mother Teresa, Dag Hammarskjold, Dietrich Bonhoeffer, Abraham Heschel, and Thomas Merton as people who reached this stage of faith development. This stage implies a radical monotheism.

Fowler's (1981) theory is not the most comprehensive of developed theory of spiritual development. Dykstra (1986) summarized the central features of Fowler's faith development theory as follows:

1    Faith is a human activity (not a thing people have, but a way of knowing and being that they are engaged in).
2    Faith is an activity that takes place through relationships.
3    The most significant aspects of these relationships are the aspects of trust and loyalty.
4    Faith involves some object(s). In faith, we trust in and are loyal to something.

5    In faith, we are related in trust and loyalty not only to persons or groups, but also to the "supra-ordinate centers of value and power" (i.e., the gods) to which people and groups whom we trust and are loyal to are also related.

6    Through these relationships of trust and loyalty our "world" (both proximate and ultimate) is shaped, meaning is made, and our own selves are constituted.

7    This activity of world-shaping, meaning-making, or "constitutive knowing" is the core activity which defines faith.

(p. 49)

## Criticism of Fowler (1981)

Parks (1992) outlined five major points of debate with Fowler's research:

They are: (1) the definition of faith; (2) the description of Stage 6; (3) the adequacy of the theory in relation to religious beliefs; (4) the adequacy of the account of affect, process, the unconscious, and the imagination, and (5) the adequacy of the theory. It is the first of these which dominate the discussion to date.

(p. 97)

Critics of Fowler (1981) have also cited the impossibility of conducting empirical research on the concepts described in the definition of faith. If the theory is comprehensive, one does not know where to begin to hypothesize. Dykstra (1986) stated that to formulate an if–then hypothesis is impossible. The definition of faith is too broad, the constructs are too vague, faith undergoes change, and some faith change is not developmental in nature. Nelson and Aleshire (1986), were critical of the research method Fowler used to develop the six stages. Stage 6 has received most of the criticisms, given that it cannot be defined and only one of nearly 400 interviewees seemed to meet Stage 6 (Broughton, 1986). Other researchers have been unable identify and measure Fowler's (1981) concepts, which are based on little research. Parks (1992) suggested that Fowler (1981) should have stopped at Stage 5 and left the rest to future research. In addition to the methodology, some questions have been posed about the reliability of the research design.

Critics have asserted that Fowler's (1981) theory is a theory of personality development, not faith development. Nelson (1992) suggested that faith development stops at adolescence and that beyond that, faith is a matter of socialization. Fernhout (1986) addressed the concept of the triadic relationship and stated that Fowler (1981) did not distinguish between faith as a way of being in relation to an ultimate environment and ways of being in relation in interpersonal and community contexts. Fowler (1981) did not define terms such as *ultimate environment* very clearly. On closer examination, however, the term means "a relationship between two points of a faith-triangle—the self and a center of value and power" (Fernhout, 1986, p. 73).

On a positive note, Parks (1992) supported Fowler's (1981) faith development theory. She stated that Fowler (1981) contributed an appealing contemporary view of faith and addressed concerns about the field of psychology. Parks (1992) made a positive analysis of the potential of Fowler's (1981) faith development theory and its relations to current theological thinking.

## Application to occupational therapy

In relation to occupational therapy, Fowler's (1981) faith theory is most appealing of the theories presented in this chapter because he believed that faith is a human universal. According to Nelson (1992), Fowler (1981) used the term *human faith* rather than *religious faith*. Nelson (1992) wrote, "Human faith to Fowler is a patterned process by which we find life meaningful. Human faith is therefore not always religious in its content or context" (p. 64). Fowler's understanding is consistent with the definition of spirituality by Seaward (2013). Fowler's (1981) idea that faith is a human concept and not a religious one can make therapists more comfortable dealing with clients who experience a spiritual crisis.

In addition, the basic tenet of Fowler's (1981) faith development accords with the concept of occupational science. Faith can be observed; it influences development, adaptation, health, quality of life and takes place in the context of culture and community. Faith is about engaging in human activity, is itself an activity, and it involves objects (Dykstra, 1986). Much of faith activity is self-care—that is taking care of the soulful self.

The idea that human faith is universal is appealing to occupational therapists because of its application to interfaith traditions. It affirms the traditional symbols, stories, and rituals of many religions and affirms that faith development can undergo transformation during the treatment process.

Concerns about clients' culture, customs, and beliefs become important considerations in treatment. Therapists are justified in supporting clients' faith traditions in the treatment process by, for example, providing time and space for Muslim clients to pray or for Buddhist clients to meditate. Educators can include the concept of faith in the occupational therapy curriculum without teaching religion or dogmatic doctrine by designing courses that encourage spiritual development among students in occupational therapy.

## Summary

This chapter reviews three theories of spiritual development; the theories of Moody and Carroll (1997), Peck (1987, 1997), and Fowler (1981). All three address the idea that people find a deep purpose in life as it unfolds in a sequence of stages. The development of faith has a slow, metamorphic effect on the adult personality. The change is called by many names, but each theorist refers to it as a conversion as the person goes from one stage to another. All seem to agree that spiritual (faith) development is not a religious concept but a universal human process.

## Active learning strategies

1 Compare and contrast two of the four theories of spiritual development. Which fits most effectively with your worldview? Why? How could this impact your therapeutic interaction with clients?
2 Write a short autobiography of yourself. Where is your spiritual development and how has it changed throughout your life? What are experiences, events, contexts which have shaped your spiritual development? How do these things influence you and your worldview as a health care provider?
3 View patient provider relationship training videos available: www. bravewell.org/integrative_medicine/educational_resources/educational_ training_videos/ examine how spirituality is or is not addressed within these training videos. Discuss with others.

## Web resources

1 Just for fun ... a quiz to examine your spiritual type: http://prayer-center. upperroom.org/resources/quiz.
2 Examine resources available at the Center for Courage and Renewal for health care providers: www.couragerenewal.org/healthcare.

## References

Assagioli, R. (1973). *The act of will.* New York: Penguin Books.
Assagioli, R. (1976). *Psychosynthesis: A collection of basic writings.* New York: Penguin Books.
Broughton, J. (1986). The political psychology of faith development theory. In C. Dykstra & S. Parks (Eds.). *Faith development and Fowler* (pp. 90–114). Birmingham, AL: Religious Education Press.
Chirban, J. (1980). *Intrinsic and extrinsic religious motivation and stages of faith* (ThD dissertation) Harvard Divinity School.
Dykstra, C. (1986). What is faith? An experiment in the hypothetical mode. In C. Dykstra & S. Parks (Eds.), *Faith development and Fowler* (pp. 45–65). Birmingham, AL: Religious Education Press.
Erikson, E. (1963). *Child and society* (2nd ed., pp. 269–274). New York: Norton.
Fernhout, H. (1986). Where is faith? Searching for the core. In C. Dykstra & S. Parks (Eds.), *Faith development and Fowler* (pp. 65–90). Birmingham, AL: Religious Education Press.
Fowler, J. (1981). *Stages of faith: The psychology of human development and the quest for meaning.* San Francisco: Harper.
Jung, C. (1957). *Modern man in search of a soul* (W. S. Dell & C. Baynes, Trans.). New York: Harvest. (Original work published 1933)

Kohlberg, L. (1968, September). The child as moral philosopher. *Psychology Today*, pp. 25–30.

Moody, H., & Carroll, D. (1997). *The five stages of the soul.* New York: Doubleday.

Nelson, C. (1992). Does faith develop? An evaluation of Fowler's position: A reader. In J. Astleu & L. Francis (Eds.), *Christian perspectives on faith development.* Grand Rapids, MI: William B. Eerdmans.

Nelson, C., & Aleshire, D. (1986). Research in faith development. In C. Dykstra & S. Parks (Eds.), *Faith development and Fowler* (pp. 180–205). Birmingham, AL: Religious Education Press.

Parks, S. (1992). Faith development in a changing world. In J. Astley & L. Francis (Eds.), *Christian perspectives on faith development* (pp. 92–107). Grand Rapids, MI: William B. Eerdmans.

Peck, S. (1987). *The different drum: Community making and peace.* New York: Simon & Schuster.

Peck, S. (1997). *The road less traveled and beyond: Spiritual growth in the age of anxiety.* New York: Simon & Schuster.

Piaget, J. (1976). *The child and reality.* New York: Penguin.

Seaward, B. (2013). *Health of the human spirit: Spiritual dimensions for personal health* (2nd ed.). London: Johns & Bartlett Learning.

# 6   Spirituality of caring

What does it really mean to say, "I really care?" Nodding (2003) states, "caring is a relationship that contains another, the cared-for, and ... the one-caring and the cared-for are reciprocally dependent" (p. 58). If an occupational therapist is having a conversation with a client and he or she cares, the therapist remains attentive in that conversation.

Caring is also viewed as a moral virtue, "as an attribute or disposition frequently exercised by a moral agent" (Nodding, 2003, p. xiii). Sometimes that moral agent is a therapist. (Caring as a moral virtue is discussed in Chapter 9.) Embedded in caring is the concept of being helpful.

People want to be helpful, but are they really? To what extent are people helpful? What percentage of the people with whom one comes in contact are helpful? And what are the ingredients of helpfulness, and why is a person not helpful? What does one need to be most helpful to the greatest number of people the largest percentage of the time? People in a helping profession need to ask themselves these questions.

To be helpful does not necessarily mean that the person is caring. Help can be given to a person out of obligation without any emotional attachment. There may be no concern about the relationship being reciprocal. The person receiving help does not have to be helpful in return. A therapist can be helpful without caring and a recipient can accept the help without forming an interactive relationship. Helpfulness is therefore necessary but not sufficient in a therapeutic environment. The therapist must be caring in order to reach a higher dimension of spiritual connection. Being helpful does not create that spiritual connection.

Mayeroff (1971) defined human caring from a secular point of view. By *secular*, he meant that the caring need have no reference to any religious experience or religious writings. He stated,

> To care for another person, in the most significant sense, is to help (that person) grow and actualize himself ... [It] is the antithesis of using the other person to satisfy one's own needs. The meaning of caring ... is not to be confused with such meanings as wishing (another person) well, liking ... or simply having an interest in what happens to another. Also, it is not an

isolated feeling or a momentary relationship, nor is it simply a matter of wanting to care for some person. Caring, as helping another grow and actualize himself, is a process, a way of relating to someone that involves development.

(p. 1)

Thus, caring is an attitude that manifests itself in concrete acts. Wanting to care and be cared for are human traits. Caring is a unifying or organizing force in human life, and caring for others and being cared for helps a person find his or her place in the world. Mayeroff (1971) stated the fundamental principle of caring as follows:

In helping the other to grow I do not impose my own direction; rather, I allow the direction of the other's growth to guide what I do, to help determine how I am to respond and what is relevant to such response. I appreciate the other as an independent in his own right with needs that are to be respected.

(p. 5)

For the therapist to impose goals, purposes, values, programs, or faith; to manipulate; or to coerce is therefore a failure to trust the basic process of human development within relationships. Caring involves an attitude and relationship as well as words and actions that produce the greatest potential for growth. The caring therapist is constantly aware that he or she is a significant part of the client's experience. The interaction between therapist and client is the total set of experiences and forms a vital part of who they are. Sharing in an open and honest way with each other is an essential part of the process of caring. Mayeroff (1971) summarized the major ingredients of caring:

- Knowledge: understanding the other person's needs and having the confidence to respond to them.
- Capacity for self-evaluation: the ability to examine the self critically and to identify behaviors that are not helpful.
- Patience: staying with the client so he or she can grow at his or her own time and pace.
- Trust: trusting the process, the relationship, and the client's own possibilities.
- Honesty: viewing oneself and the other as they really are and not as one wants to view them. It is critical that client and therapist see each other as they actually are.
- Humility: never thinking one knows all there is to know about oneself and the other; recognizing that there are limitations and that there is always something more to learn.
- Hope: having hope about what will happen to and for the other person as a result of the caring.

• Courage: understanding that there is always a risk, because one involves the self without knowing the outcome. Caring people invest a part of themselves, their knowledge, their skills, and their hope. Courage is going into the unknown with another.

## Therapeutic use of self and caring

A caring person is in constant pursuit of knowledge about the self. Knowing the self is consistent with the concept of the therapeutic use of self. In the therapeutic environment, to interact in community with another person, it is important to have knowledge about the self and about the techniques of therapy. Therapists can assume that the clients they see in the clinic are there as a result of grief or loss and are experiencing a spiritual crisis. The term *spiritual crisis* or *spiritual distress* describes a pervasive disruption in a person's spiritual life (Hasselkus, 2002) resulting from injury or disease. When the body is threatened, attacked, or in the process of debilitation and malfunction, the person experiences a situation that may manifest as fear and anxiety. Often, people regress to a time when they felt safe and free from pain. This mental process leaves them somewhat helpless and unable to function in the usual way. A person confined to bed, for example, has had to withdraw from meaningful activities and contact with family, friends, and the community and therefore will feel a sense of loss. If the person is hospitalized, he or she is separated from the physical environment and perceives a threat to his or her body and, thus, to the self. For many people, these losses include their community of faith and the worship and other activities to which they are accustomed. Their participation in the life of worshiping is lost.

Hay (1989) listed the characteristics of spiritual crisis as follows:

• Pain, constant and chronic
• Insomnia
• Withdrawal or isolation from one's spiritual support system
• Conflict with family members, friends, or support staff
• Anxiety; fear; and mistrust of family, friends, physicians, and hospice staff
• Anger
• Depression
• Guilt, low-self-worth, and comments about self-loathing
• Hopelessness
• Feeling of failure with life
• Lack of a sense of humor
• Lack of forgiveness
• Despair
• Fear and dread.

(p. 27)

Hay (1989) also stated that religion can contribute to spiritual pain when people foster guilt or a sense of condemnation or rejection (from God or the faith community). Religious doctrines of eternal judgment and discouragement of the process of an individualized search for meaning (including the expression of painful feelings and difficult questions) can cause spiritual pain, and the client can enter a spiritual crisis.

When the client is first referred to an occupational therapy department, the therapist needs to remember that the client is coming from a community made up of a biological family, a work family, a faith family, and any other group that is a part of his or her lifestyle and life space. These groups are subject to systems theory that contains a worldview. Systems involve work, emotion, and life stories and are designed to sustain a set of values. These groups have life stories that involve a set of values that represent a worldview.

A set of values involves relationships that can be centered on listening to one another's stories. When developing a relationship through listening to stories, the client is responding to four voices in his or her consciousness (Moseley, 2008):

1  *Voices from the present*: When clients are being challenged by something they need to acknowledge, they must examine what they are valuing. Are they trying to change this value? Are they working to accept a new value? This process can cause anxiety. Some voices come from religious institutions that influence behavior and thinking—church, synagogue, temple, or mosque, for example.
2  *Voices from the past*: These voices, such as those of parents and teachers, tell the client how to behave. The therapist is listening to the meaning behind the client's words. These voices are always present, and they are more powerful than the therapist's. These voices are from the past and give messages about religious beliefs and the concept of prayer.
3  *Voices from the culture*: The culture is the sum of the beliefs, practices, habits, likes, dislikes, norms, customs, and rituals that one learns from the family during the years of socialization. The culture shapes how the client hears, and it is loud. It molds the person's attitude and can be full of subconscious voices. The client usually is not aware of where the voices come from. Sometimes they are from the past, which is where anger and shame come from. To know where the voices come from is to understand oneself and one's pain.
4  *Voices from the future*: These voices are heard from the therapist in response to the client's stories, in answers to questions in an interview, and in messages that are given in the interaction. Responses that have implications for the future are always initiated in the present.

During the treatment process, the client is in crisis and is challenged to explore the nature of the voices. The voices he or she hears are coming from the external world and from the past, and the therapist is bringing voices from the future.

The client is being encouraged to develop new systems or a worldview that will be more productive and help him or her to become healthy.

Everyone has a group of four voices that create a sense of stability. It is important to physically stay with clients as they express anxiety and other emotions about their disability. The caring person does not take away those feelings by denying them or minimizing them in any way. Rather, it is essential that the therapist allows and sometimes assists clients with expressing their pain, anguish, and other feelings. To deal with another's intense anger, the caring person needs to be able to deal with his or her own anger. Otherwise, he or she will be ineffective or change the subject.

## Facilitative conditions of spiritual relationships

One of the guiding principles of the therapeutic use of self is the importance of self-care and knowledge of the self. Knowing the divine self is the central theme in a relationship—the caring relationship *is* the divine self. When sharing his or her innermost thoughts, a person is vulnerable. Certain conditions foster a spiritual relationship that is authentic and transparent and that meets the client's needs. Authors such as Carkhuff (1969), Egan (1990), and Okun (1992) have made suggestions about what facilitates the development of spiritual relationships that will meet the needs of clients who are in crisis. The following human characteristics are important in occupational therapy practice and will enhance the use of self and establish a spiritual relationship.

### *Empathy*

Empathy involves identifying with clients by assuming their frame of reference. The desired outcome is to foster trust in the relationship-centered care (RCC) described in Chapter 4, to communicate understanding, and to encourage deeper levels of self-exploration (Corey & Corey, 1993). In being understood, the client experiences comfort, hope, and a movement into a state in which faith has the greatest possibility of being stimulated. The caring person does not give hope, faith, assurance, and comfort but provides the conditions within which the other person is most likely to experience them (Switzer, 2000). According to Switzer (2000), "the power of growth for the other is not in our understanding, but in the person's experience of being understood" (p. 23). Active listening is the beginning point for empathy.

### *Respect*

Respect is important in a spiritual crisis in that the client feels as though he or she is a worthwhile human being as the result of the caring therapist's investment. The word *respect* comes from a Latin root (*vereor*) that includes the notion of seeing or viewing; respect is a particular way of viewing oneself and others. It means prizing people simply because they are human. Characteristics of respect for clients are as follows:

- *Do no harm*: Clients should not be manipulated into a lifestyle selected by the caring person.
- *Treat patients as individuals*: Prize the client as an individual, and support his or her search for the divine self.
- *Suspend critical judgment*: This kind of respect is called *unconditional positive regard* (Rogers, 1961).
- *Be for the client*: Act as the client's advocate.
- *Be available*: Be available in a reasonable way.
- *Understand and communicate understanding to clients*: People understand that they are respected if the caring person takes the time and effort to understand them.
- *Assume the client's goodwill*: Work on the assumption that clients want to live more effectively with their disability.
- *Be warm within reason*: Clients look for competence, experience, a good reputation, and warmth in their caring person.
- *Help clients use their own resources*: The caring person's attitude is that clients have resources with which to manage their life. Respect means helping clients use their resources effectively so that they can participate fully in the relationship-centered relationship.
- *Help clients through the pain*: Respect includes the assumption that the client is willing to pay the price of living more effectively. The caring person places demands but helps the client meets those demands.

### Concreteness

Concreteness is a prerequisite to effective empathy. It means speaking simply and with clarity. It means asking questions about what expressions or words mean and what feelings a person is referring to. It also means encouraging more detail and requesting illustrations. This interaction strips away the ego so that people meet on the level of soulfulness. The therapist cannot express empathy unless he or she can be assured of the client's feelings, what the client's experience is like, and what the client is thinking.

### Self-disclosure

It is important in the relationship-centered relationship for the caring person to be known as a human being. The caring person is not just the position that he or she holds but is a helping person. Sometimes, if only for a moment, it can be useful for the caring person to share with the client a feeling or experience of confusion or pain. The caring person could also share his or her convictions, meanings, or faith. Therapists must be careful about how facts and factors are expressed. The caring person should not call attention to himself or herself, coerce or manipulate the client into aligning with the caring person's religious tradition, or force advice onto the client. Self-disclosure is effective when it is brief and attention is turned immediately back to the client.

## Confrontation

In a caring relationship, one often finds inconsistencies between what one says and what one does. The difference in expressions of words and behavior is known as a *discrepancy*. The caring person therefore listens for inconsistencies. At a well-timed point in the relationship, when the client can deal with the stress and is understood sufficiently, the caring person confronts the client with the inconsistency. Switzer (2000) stated that confrontation "is a type of crisis for the person, a discrepancy between self-image and behavior, goals and behavior, faith and behavior, our real feelings and how we would like to present ourselves" (p. 30). Confrontation, however, is an opportunity for the client to grow and experience honest feedback about his or her behavior.

## Immediacy

Egan (1990) identified two types of immediacy: *relationship immediacy* and *here-and-now immediacy*. The first type is the caring person's ability to discuss where the client stands with the relationship. The focus is on the way in which the relationship itself has developed. The second type of immediacy is the caring person's ability to discuss with the client what is happening between the client and caring person in the "here and now." It does not include the entire relationship, just what is happening in a specific situation. Egan (1990) gave the following example:

> The therapist uses self-disclosure and here-and-now immediacy to focus on a key issue in the patient's interpersonal life. She begins to explore the possibility that what the patient is doing here and now is an example of his self-defeating approach to interpersonal relationships in his everyday life.
>
> (p. 227)

## Pragmatism

The caring person can express pragmatism in a variety of ways (Egan, 1990):

- Keep the client's agenda in focus: Pursue the client's agenda, not one's own.
- Maintain a real-life focus: Help clients manage their day-to-day life more effectively.
- Continue to learn: Be a lifelong learner.
- Use modeling: Model behavior that one wants one's client to learn.
- Be assertive: If the therapist is good at what he or she does, he or she should be proud and not apologize for it.
- Find competence not in behavior, but in outcomes.

Pragmatism enables the therapist to be more concerned with practical results than with theories and occupational therapy principles. Being pragmatic emphasizes the need to learn from the client. The teacher becomes the learner.

## Genuineness

*Genuineness* refers to a set of attitudes and a set of therapist behaviors. To some people, being genuine means being congruent. It can also mean being comfortable with oneself (Egan, 1990). Being comfortable means knowing one's spirituality and being able to relate on a spiritual level.

- Do not overemphasize the importance of caring role. Caring persons should learn how to listen without distorting what they hear.
- Be spontaneous, and avoid defensiveness.
- Be consistent and open.
- Work at becoming comfortable with behavior that helps clients.

Okun (1992) listed the following additional therapist characteristics that are consistent with effectiveness: self-awareness, gender and cultural awareness, honesty, knowledge, and ethical integrity.

## Self-awareness

Self-awareness can result in more effective use of the self as a vehicle to promote change in the client. Self-aware people are more likely to be able to separate their perceived needs and feelings from those of the client. Self-awareness is a developmental process, and self-aware therapists can experience the client's pain and anxiety and the impact on culture and familial influences. In addition, self-aware therapists are more likely to help clients develop self-awareness.

## Gender and cultural awareness

Therapists who are sensitive to the influence of gender and culture on perceptions, values, attitudes, and religious beliefs are open to the effects of these phenomena on health and wellness. Therapists need to know how to modify and adapt to non-Western ways of health care beyond the set of caring behaviors specific to Western culture.

## Honesty

When a caring person is open, answers questions to the best of his or her ability, and admits mistakes or lack of knowledge, he or she is being honest.

## Knowledge

Professional helpers should have knowledge about the current research on psychological theory, normal and abnormal development, neuropsychology, personality, and gender development. The therapist should be knowledgeable about sociological theory, about roles and influences of culture on people's development and behavior. The study of multicultural, sexual orientation, and gender is an addition to the academic training of therapist. Empirically based and evidence-based treatment are terms increasingly needed to deliver mental health services.

### *Ethical integrity*

Ethical integrity overlaps with honesty and congruence. It involves a conscious effort on the part of the therapist to behave responsibly, morally, and ethically. The therapist has to decide what behaviors are responsible, moral, and ethical; engage in self-reflection; and make continued efforts to understand the client's cultural, ethnic, and religious traditions. The therapist must cope every day with ambiguity, uncertainty, and ambivalence about complex and challenging ethical dilemmas. The ethics of caring are addressed further in Chapter 9.

## Prayer as a form of caring

A caring person is concerned with the client's spiritual life. Prayerfulness has become a predictor of well-being, and it produces relaxation. Prayer has a positive psychophysical effect on the immune system. According to Dossey (1993), "the term prayer comes from the Latin *precarious*, 'obtained by begging,' and *precari*, 'to entreat'—to ask earnestly, beseech, implore" (p. 5). There are prayers of petition, intercession, confession, lamentation, adoration, invocation, and thanksgiving. In occupational therapy, prayer is a performance component that expresses a person's religious tradition. Making the therapeutic environment conducive to a prayerful atmosphere communicates a caring and respectful attitude (Dossey, 1993).

Praying with a client is becoming more acceptable (Dossey, 1993). Even so, many people would not ask their therapist to pray with them. Accordingly, the therapist can take one of three approaches with regard to praying with people: (1) Never do it, (2) always do it, or (3) make the decision on the basis of one's best judgment about the client, and the situation. When the client asks to pray with the therapist, it is important that the therapist knows him or her well enough. If he or she does not know the client well, clues from prior conversations, such as references to the client's faith tradition or prayer life, church relationship, and other language of faith, can give information that can be included in the prayer. The therapist loses nothing by asking whether the client would like to pray unless the client has given the therapist sufficient clues that he or she wants nothing to do with anything like that. It is preferable for the client to do the praying and the therapist to participate in the act of prayer. The prayer by the therapist, however, must be in the context of the client's faith tradition. When the client's faith tradition is not the same as the therapist's, and the therapist is uncomfortable with it, praying should be referred to another therapist.

Rosenfeld (2000) offered steps for crafting prayers. He emphasized that clients must identify a name for their creator or universal force; select a focus for their prayer; and can include prayers of praise, thanksgiving, and petition. Rosenfeld (2000) stated, "Learning to craft prayers can improve performance skills in self-awareness and expression, art, poetry, music, worship, and personal goal setting" (p. 19). It is acceptable to use the client's sacred literature, such as the Torah, Koran, or Bible. At the beginning of the session, the therapist should develop an atmosphere of reverence—for example, by introducing inspirational music and beginning with a reading from a secular source (see Appendix A). If the client is not religious, there is no reason to participate in spiritual activities. However, the therapist should encourage or facilitate the client's spiritual practice.

Prayer can take many forms. Some people pray to a personal god or goddess, the almighty, or a supreme being; others pray to an impersonal universe or the absolute; and still others do not pray in any conventional sense but live deeply and have a sense of the sacred. This kind of prayer is called a *spirit of prayerfulness*, wherein people are attuned to something greater than themselves. Western types of prayer use structure and follow instructions; prayerfulness does not. It involves a feeling of unity with the All and has no attachment to religious leaders, traditions, or holy books. Dossey (1993) stated, "Prayerfulness … is accepting without being passive, is grateful without giving up. It is more willing to stand in the mystery, to tolerate ambiguity and the unknown. It honors the rightness of whatever happens" (p. 24).

There is no guarantee that clients will experience freedom from illness. They can, however, achieve wellness. This wellness could be a placebo effect, the therapist's initial action might have had a real but delayed effect, the therapist may continue to pray for the client outside the treatment setting, or the therapist's belief may somehow have an effect on the client's improvement. There is no cause and effect relationship between prayer and wellness. However, the client as well as the therapist must believe that the prayer is effective. If the therapist believes in prayer, it is appropriate to use it at a distance without the client present. Prayer and belief are related; similarly, the therapist should never select a therapy technique that he or she believes will not work. The therapist should never be unnecessarily pessimistic and should be as hopeful and open as possible.

Occupational therapists need not be chameleons and offer prayers from religious traditions different from their own. Rather, they should participate in clients' own prayer traditions or give opportunities for clients to do so. If a prayer is beyond the skills of a therapist, he or she must search for a suitable professional for assistance. The following sections are intended to make occupational therapists aware of the differences among prayer traditions.

## Prayer in the context of Christianity

Moore-Keish (2009) stated that "it is good to acknowledge what Christian prayers have in common with the prayers of other religious traditions. Of course, not all religious traditions include prayers" (pp. 37–38). Christians are not the only faith "that sit, kneel, or prostrate themselves before God. We are not the only ones who light candles, whisper or chant, or shout praise and petitions to a power greater than ourselves" (Moore-Keish, 2009, p. 38). Prayers are not all alike. Christian prayers are distinctive, because Christian prayers end with the words "in the name of Jesus" (Moore-Keish, 2009, p. 38). If there is anything that distinguishes Christian prayers it is these words. These words are not just a tagline but the "foundation, goal and resting place in which we offer our prayer" (Moore-Keish, 2009, p. 39). *Lord Jesus Christ, Son of God, have mercy on me, a sinner* is a prayer known as the "Jesus Prayer." It is one example of praying in "the name of Jesus" (Moore-Keish, 2009, p. 39).

The context of prayer can be in secret, in families, in communities, and public (sometimes called cooperate) prayer. There is the belief in God. Moore-Kiesh (2009) and Pearce (2003) listed several kinds of prayers:

- *Adoration*: "This mode of prayer attends particularly to God as the one whom we address, the transcendent One to whom our prayers are directed" (Moore-Keish, 2009, p. 61).
- *Confession*: The honest telling of one's sins and mistakes to God (Pearce, 2003, p. ix).
- *Thanksgiving*: Prayers of thanksgiving not only express our gratitude for such gifts; over time, such prayers can also shape us into fundamentally grateful people (Moore-Keish, 2009, p. 63). "Bonhoeffer says, '[W]e need to do this not only alone and not only in community, but with another member of the Christian community' " (p. 62).
- *Petition (supplication) and intercession*: Some people believe that God really answers prayers. Prayers that ask "God's intervening grace, either for themselves (supplication, petition) or for others (intercession)" are in this category (Moore-Keish, 2009, p. 64).
- *Invocation*: is "the intentional reminding of oneself that God is present, the awareness of the Divine presence" (Pearce, 2003, p. viii).
- *Lament*: "In adoration we cry out to God." Lamentation is crying out to God "in our anguish" (Moore-Keish, 2009, p. 66).

Prayer can be carried by means other than words. It can be present in all the senses, including the body. It can be expressed in dance, breathing, visual arts, silence, and music. Prayer can be conversational—with another person or with the transcendent being. Christian prayer is the "chief exercise of faith" (Moore-Keish, 2009, p. 79).

## Prayer in the context of Islam

Muslims face Mecca (i.e., east) and pray five times a day for *Salah*. In the context of Islam, each opening prayer is repeated in the Muslim's five daily prayers. Prayers are offered in Arabic, the language of Muhammad. An example of an opening prayer is as follows:

In the Name of Allah the Merciful, the Compassionate:
Praise be to Allah, Creator of the worlds,
The Merciful, the Compassionate,
Ruler of the day of Judgment.
Thee do we worship, and Thee do we ask for aid.
Guide us in the straight path,
The path of those on whom Thou hast poured forth Thy grace.
Not the path of those who have incurred Thy wrath and gone astray.

(Huston, 1991, p. 243)

The straight path is straightforward and direct; it spells out how Muslims must live. The contents of this path are the five pillars of Islam: (1) the confession of faith, (2) canonical prayer, (3) charity, (4) observance of Ramadan, and (5) pilgrimage. The canonical prayer is to be faithful and constant. The reason Muslims pray five times is twofold: (1) to give thanks for God's presence, and (2) to keep life in perspective and stay on the straight and narrow. The essence of prayer comes down to submitting to the will of God. The times of prayer are stipulated in the Koran: on rising, when the sun reaches its zenith, when the sun reaches its midline, at sunset, and before retiring. Muslims are expected to pray in mosques when they can and always on Friday; noon prayer is the most important.

Before prayer, it is important that Muslims wash their body, to symbolically wash their soul. This ritual is call *wudu.* The practice is a ritual purification rather than a matter of hygiene. No soap is used, and when water is unavailable one can simply go through the motions of washing with one's dry hands. After entering the state of ritual purity, the Muslim stands facing Mecca and makes the formal intention to pray. *Salat* prayers consist of a set of Koranic verses that are recited in a cycle of standing, sitting, and kneeling positions. Each cycle is called a *raks.* In prayer, the person sinks and touches his or her forehead to the floor (Huston, 1991). This is the prayer's holiest moment. The body is in a fetal position, symbolizing rebirth, and at the same time is in the smallest possible space, which symbolizes "nothingness in the face of the divine" (Huston, 1991, p. 246). The contents of the prayer are praise, gratitude, and supplication. A *salat* "prayer is not prayer in the sense of a personal conversation with God, but rather a ritual obligation which must be fulfilled to reaffirm one's relationship with God" (Elias, 1999, pp. 66–67).

A caring person respects others' faith traditions. In working with Muslim clients, the therapist needs to remember to make prayer possible and to indicate which way is east. The therapist should integrate the times of prayer into the treatment process and provide the means to wash before prayer. When it is impossible for the client to prostrate on the floor, the therapist should adapt the place of prayer to the client's needs by making it possible to get onto the floor.

## Prayer in the context of Judaism

Jews recite the Biblical psalms and other traditional prayers, especially on holy days, such as Rosh Hashanah and Yom Kippur. Many Jews lead a prayerful life and pray daily in ways that are as individual as the communities in which they live (Emmons, 2006). At the heart of Jewish prayer is the idea that God listens to prayer and that prayer is a dialogue between a person and his or her creator. The variety of prayers in the Jewish liturgy suggests the many faceted nature of the relationship between God and humanity. In the course of a single service, prayers may mention "God the Creator, the Redeemer, the Father, the Judge, Rock of Israel, Shield of Abraham, and many others. Each of these personifications of God implies a different relationship between the Deity and the person praying" (Robinson, 2000, p. 8).

It is possible for Jewish patients to pray alone, but it is preferable that prayers be offered in a communal setting (*not a minyan*). Praying in a community serves many functions. It helps people deal with an environment that is chaotic, arbitrary, and indecipherable. It gives great comfort during times of crisis when people who are praying are surrounded by like-minded worshipers. During a health crisis, it is preferable that Jewish patients be treated together in the therapeutic environment whenever possible.

In addition, while in the therapeutic setting, the patient's worship community should participate in any worship service as though the patient were in his or her home. The prayer rituals are designed to reinforce the sense of community and to give a feeling of being tied to a historical continuity. Robinson (2000) noted that "the complex web of relationships between the individual Jew, the worship community, and the Jewish people, between past and present, is an essential part of the Jewish experience of communal prayer" (p. 14) while in a health facility. A study of the sacred text (the Torah) is considered to be an integral part of the worship. It is important that the therapist makes available Jewish texts if the client does not have his or her own.

In Orthodox Judaism, women pray in an atmosphere of silence and do not participate in communal prayer. They are not required to attend a public place of worship. It is important that the occupational therapist be aware of the order of service so that he or she can make necessary adaptations. In the Jewish worship service, the regular Orders of Service are recited. They are *Maariv* (or *Aravit*) in the evening, *Shacharit* in the morning, and *Mincha* in the afternoon. The two major prayers in the Jewish faith are the *Shema*, which consists of three scriptural readings and opens with the declaration of God's unity, and the *Amida* or *Shemone Esreh*, which consists of prayers of praise, petitions, and thanksgiving (Solomon, 2000). Worshipers say the *Amida* prayer quietly, standing reverently, facing Jerusalem; at four points they bow slightly. Concentration is more important than bodily position. When a person is sick enough that standing would interfere with concentration, sitting is permitted. As the prayer begins, the person commits to the unity of God in the first verse ("Hear, O Israel! The Lord is our God. The Lord is One!"). The person stays still, with eyes closed in intense concentration. Deuteronomy 6:4–9 of the Torah is recited (Solomon, 2000). If the person is too agitated to assume a prayerful attitude, it should not be attempted. Jewish praying in the context of worshiping can be very public and distracting to other clients if it is done in a communal setting. Conducting silent prayer on a one-to-one basis is preferred.

## Prayer in the context of Buddhism

Buddhism is most prevalent in the countries of China, Japan, and Korea, and in Southeast Asia. There are generally two types of Buddhism: the Theravada and the Mahayana. The Theravada practices meditation, and the Mahayana includes petitionary prayer (Huston, 1991). Generally, Buddhists' central religious practice is meditation. It should not be considered equivalent of prayer. Buddhists seek to awaken a source of spiritual power from within themselves. This is called "the Buddha-nature within" (Bickel & Jantz, 2002). Mahayana Buddhists pray daily to attain oneness with the ultimate power. Meditation is the form of prayer. Prayers may occur out loud, but people often simply meditate on a *mantra*, or sacred utterance. The most famous mantra is the "Om Mani Pedme Hum" (Snelling, 1991). This mantra is inscribed on flags, painted on walls, twirled within prayer wheels, and even carved on stones and wayside rocks. It is literally translated as "Hail to the jewel in the lotus."

Stephan Batchelor (1984) wrote that the mantra "functions as a symbolic and highly condensed expression of the entire path to enlightenment" (p. 170). It is a word or phrase that is repeated countless times until the mind is cleared of all else. Noise is converted into sound and distracting chatter into holy formulas (Huston, 1991). A mantra is eternal and uncreated, divine power itself in the form of sound. Chanting a mantra puts the believer into an intimate relationship with the divine (Emmons, 2006). Snelling (1991) stated, "Recitation of a mantra represents a kind of practice that can be readily carried on in everyday situations. It purifies the speech and 'protects the mind' by maintaining a constant spiritual connection; and ... it helps disperse mental chatter" (p. 96).

Mantras are highly compressed, power-packed formulas, usually of Sanskrit origin, that are charged with deep meaning and magical potency. The belief that certain natural sounds in themselves are mantras is common among Tibetan Buddhists. They carve mantras on prayer wheels and fly prayer flags to carry their prayers to the winds. Emmons (2006) stated, "Hindus also meditate using mantras, but they also pray before icons representing what they believe to be incarnations of God—Brahma, Vishnu, and Siva" (p. 13). A caring therapist is aware of these forms of prayer and allows the symbolism to be used in the therapeutic setting.

During meditation, the person assumes a cross-legged posture or a sitting position (Soto Zen tradition). The cross-legged posture is the classic position. It can be with one leg laid on top of the other or it can be two legs interwoven. If either gives pain to the client a chair may be used. The back is straight unsupported and the hips are slightly tilted forward. The head should be upright, the eyelids lowered and the mouth lightly closed. The hands are laid one on top of the other with the thumbs lightly touching. There is also a form of walking, and in extreme cases the client can be lying down (Snelling, 1991). He or she lays aside all personal problems and preoccupations and uses specialized techniques. According to Snelling (1991), Carl Jung observed mandalic patterns of thought and dreams among patients, which he saw as tokens of spiritual paths. Therapists must recognize mantras as legitimate spiritual practice. *Mandala* is a sacred space where the person sets out on a spiritual journey through contemplation to awaken latent spiritual material deep in the subconscious. The therapist should give the client the space and opportunity to meditate and use whatever symbols are appropriate. In basic Buddhist meditation, two elements are usually identified: *Shamatha* (in Pali, *Samatha*), literally, "calm abiding," and *Vipashyana* (in Pali, *Vipassana*), or insight. In shamatha there is concentration on a single object such as breath or sensations of the body. Vipashyana is a deeper form of meditation where insight is analyzed and observed (Snelling, 1991).

The meditating person concentrates on a single object to the exclusion of all others. The object may be breath, a colored disk, or the sensations of the body, but it should be neutral, unexciting, and invocative. Complete concentration is necessary for vipashyana to be reached. The mind is opened, and awareness is directed to all that enters its sphere. During this phase, psychological material may arise into consciousness. Old fears and phobias, traumas, and repressions come to full awareness. The therapist needs to be cognizant of this possibility. When the client's mind quiets down, attention may be directed in a more systematic way. The therapist needs to give the client his or her sacred space and provide privacy and whatever is possible to assist the client.

As the mind quiets down and meditation is occurring, the client reaches a state of mindfulness. Four states of mindfulness occur when the client focuses.

There are four foundations of mindfulness:

1   Bodily activity
2   Feelings
3   States of mind
4   Mental contents.

(Snelling, 1991, pp. 52–53)

Whatever enters the field of attention is observed and analyzed. Buddhism does not ask such questions as "Who made the world?" "What is the meaning of life?" or "What happens to us after death?" It is not concerned with the question of the existence of a god or gods. It examines the "I." The self is a delusion; the ultimate mystery is the divine self. Snelling (1991) wrote that

> the mystery is at the heart of all things, and confronts what the Christians call God, the Muslims Allah, the Hindus Brahman. Buddhists … hesitate to put a name to it. It is … something that cannot be grasped by the intellect or described in words.
>
> (p. 7)

## Prayer in the context of Native American faith

Meditation is not unique to Buddhism. There are 10 large American Indian nations in the United States. All of them practice a form of meditation, sometimes in the form of a "vision quest." Native Americans use vision quests to meditate with nature, awaiting a clear vision of life's purpose. Dallas Chief Eagle stated that a "vision quest teaches one simplicity, humility, and it certainly adjusts one's attitudes in a spiritual way" (Steiger, 1984, p. 33). In the Judea-Christian tradition, Isaac, Abraham, and Jacob can be said to have gone on vision quests. The seeker goes into the wilderness alone to receive a guardian spirit and a secret name. In the Native American faith, this process is essential if one is to receive the essence of medicine power.

*Medicine power* is the ability to "obtain personal contact with the invisible world of spirits and to pierce the sensory world of illusion which veils the great mystery" (Steiger, 1984, p. 25). One of the essential elements of medicine power is the vision quest, with its "emphasis on self-denial and spiritual discipline, extended to a lifelong pursuit of wisdom of body and soul" (Steiger, 1984, p. 31). The tradition of the vision quest places an emphasis on individualism and sacredness of personal vision, and it results in a mystical experience. It is referred to as the *mesquakie tradition* (vision quest). People believe in the vision quest because the experience affirms the belief in a higher being that tells one what to do, "to tell ... the way to help one's people, help the family, and help the tribe" (Steiger, 1984, p. 34).

The vision quest is basic to all native North American religious experience. Young men and women embark on a vision quest at an early age and consider it to be their "first communion" (Steiger, 1984, p. 36). To a Catholic child, a first communion could feel like a coming-of-age experience. It marks the beginning of a lifelong search for knowledge and wisdom. Obtaining a guardian spirit is important, for this spirit guides and shapes the person's destiny. Steiger (1984) wrote that in "any stress period of his/her life, the traditional American Indian may go into the wilderness to fast and to seek insight into the particular problems that beset him" (p. 36). The Native American faith makes the vision quest a part of the life of everyone who seeks medicine power. Those who embark on the vision quest treat the guardian spirit with respect and use the information given in dreams and visions as lessons to be drawn on in the performance of their personal medicine. The meditative state is achieved during the vision quest, and meditation is the door into silence, where the person can communicate with his or her inner self and the spiritual energy.

In a rehabilitative environment, whether it be for physical rehabilitation or mental health, the therapist must be aware of the concept of vision quests and be willing to listen to dreams. Asking clients to record and discuss their dreams is an important role of the therapist. Therapists need to be aware of their own dreams and be willing to discuss them with the client, because dreams are universal and can be intertwined with the client's dreams. The client needs to be given physical space in the clinic (perhaps a corner in the clinic) and time during the treatment process to engage in vision quests. The therapist should respect and discuss the results of the person's quest so that the insight can be integrated into the treatment process. Finally, in prayer, a traditional Native American never asks and never offers prayers of supplication; he or she makes only prayers of thanksgiving.

# Summary

A prayerful atmosphere is one of caring, and praying is a universal phenomenon. A therapist who encounters various cultures in the treatment setting will come in contact with various methods of praying. He or she should respect those methods and integrate them into the treatment process when necessary.

Therapists can express a caring attitude through the therapeutic use of self by using empathy, respect, concreteness, self-disclosure, confrontation, immediacy, pragmatism, genuineness, self-awareness, gender and cultural awareness, honesty, and ethical integrity. A therapist who is able to enhance the treatment process with a caring attitude will increase his or her chances for success.

Finally, Steiger (1984) reported that healers all over the world use four common components of curing:

- *Naming process*—Naming the ailment, complaint, or illness that fits with the patient's worldview may help generate wellness.
- *Personal characteristics of the healer*—Personal qualities of accurate empathy, nonpossessive warmth, and genuineness achieve better results.
- *Patient's expectations*—Amulets, rattles, stethoscopes, or diplomas are common ways to increase expectations. It has been observed that the farther the patient has to travel to see the healer, the more the chances of wellness increase.
- *The healer's training*—Some cultures do not have examinations after training, as do Western cultures. All over the world, however, cultures require rigorous training programs for healers that may last several years.

(p. 55)

Occupational therapists should respect these characteristics and remember them as universal. Readers are reminded that the best information about how a vision quest is carried out is to consult with the client and make the necessary arrangements in the clinic. If the specific tribe member does not practice vision quests, it is important not to make judgments about their spiritual practices. Their spiritual practices may be Westernized and consistent with other faith traditions.

# References

Batchelor, S. (1984). The jewel and the lotus: A survey of the Buddhism of Tibet. *Middle Way, 3*(59), 170–175.

Bickel, B. & Jantz, S. (2002). *World Religions & Cults 101*. Eugene, OR: Harvest House Publishers.

Carkhuff, R. (1969). *Helping and human relations* (Vols. 1 & 2). New York: Holt, Rinehart & Winston.

Corey, M., & Corey, G. (1993). *Becoming a helper.* Pacific Grove, CA: Brooks/Cole.

Dossey, L. (1993). *Healing words: The power of prayer and the practice of medicine.* San Francisco: HarperSanFrancisco.

Egan, G. (1990). *The skilled helper: A systematic approach to effective helping.* Pacific Grove, CA: Brooks/Cole.

Elias, J. (1999). *Islam.* Upper Saddle River, NJ: Prentice Hall.

Emmons, S. (2006). The world prays. *Disciples World, 5*(10), 13–15.

Hasselkus, B. (2002). *The meaning of everyday occupation.* Thorofare, NJ: Slack.

Hay, M. W. (1989). Principles in building spiritual assessment tools. *American Journal of Hospice Care, 6*(5), 25–31.

Huston, S. (1991). *The world religions: Our great wisdom traditions.* New York: HarperCollins.

Mayeroff, M. (1971). *On caring.* New York: Harper & Row.

Moore-Keish, M. L. (2009). *Christian prayer for today.* Louisville, KY: Westminster John Knox Press.

Moseley, D. (2008). *Living with loss.* Nashville, TN: Xyzzy Press.

Nodding, N. (2003). *Caring: A feminine approach to ethics and moral education.* Berkeley: University of California Press.

Okun, B. (1992). *Effective helping.* Belmont, CA: Brooks/Cole.

Pearce, M. K. (2003). *Concerning prayer.* New York: General Board of Global Ministries.

Robinson, G. (2000). *Essential Judaism: A complete guide to beliefs, customs, and rituals.* New York: Pocket Books.

Rogers, C. (1961). *On becoming a person.* Boston: Houghton Mifflin.

Rosenfeld, M. (2000, January 17). Spiritual agent modalities for occupational therapy practice. *OT Practice*, pp. 17–21.

Snelling, J. (1991). *The Buddhist handbook: A complete guide to Buddhist schools, teaching, practice, and history.* New York: Barnes & Noble.

Solomon, N. (2000). *Judaism: A very short introduction.* New York: Oxford University Press.

Steiger, B. (1984). *Indian medicine power.* Atglen, PA: Whitford Press.

Switzer, D. (2000). *Pastoral care emergencies.* Minneapolis, MN: Fortress Press.

# 7 Spiritual and cultural diversity in the occupational therapy clinic

Spirituality is expressed in the culture of the individual through their worldview. Through art, media, dress, food, and religious rituals and customs the individual's spirituality is realized. The therapist is advised to be aware of the cultural practices that affect the delivery of health care that enhances patients' spirituality. This chapter is a brief outline of cultural practices that influence occupational therapy practice.

Culture care is a term coined by Spector (2000) to describe professional health care that is culturally sensitive, culturally appropriate, and culturally competent. It demands that the therapist be able to assess and interpret a given patient's health beliefs and practices. Spector stated that "cultural care alters the perspective of health-care delivery as it enables the provider to understand, from a cultural perspective, the manifestations of the patient's health-care beliefs and practices" (p. 281). According to Spector (p. 79):

- Culture is the medium of personhood and social relationships.
- Culture is conscious.
- Culture can be likened to a prosthetic device because it is an extension of biological capabilities.
- Culture is an interlinked web of symbols.
- Culture is a device for creating and limiting human choices.
- Culture can be in two places at once—it is found in a person's mind and also exists in the environment in such form as the spoken word or an artifact.

Culture is the sum of beliefs, practices, habits, likes, dislikes, norms, customs, and rituals that are learned from our families during the years of socialization. Cultural background is a fundamental component of one's ethnic background. Ethnicity is not the same as culture. "Ethnicity is that part of one's identity derived from membership, usually through birth, in a racial, religious, national, or linguistic group or subgroup" (Krefting, 2003, p. 203). Ethnicity is indicative of the following characteristics that a group may share in some combination (p. 81):

- Common geographic origin.
- Migratory status.

- Race.
- Language and dialect.
- Religious faith or faiths.
- Ties that transcend kinship, neighborhood, and community boundaries.
- Shared traditions, values, and symbols.
- Literature, folklore, and music.
- Food preferences.
- Settlement and employment patterns.
- Special interest with regard to politics in the homeland and in the United States.

Giger and Davidhizar (1995) have identified six cultural phenomena that vary among cultural groups and affect health care. They are:

- Environmental control. This is the ability to plan activities that control nature or direct environmental factors. Included are concepts of traditional health and illness beliefs, such as the practice of vision quests, folk medicine, and the use of traditional healers. The use of health healers influences the way patients respond to health-related experiences including health care resources and social supports.
- Biological variations. People from one culture group differ biologically from other culture groups. Differences can involve bodily build; skin color, including variations in tone, texture, and healing abilities; enzymatic and genetic variations, including differences in response to drug and dietary therapies; and susceptibility to disease, which can manifest itself in a higher morbidity rate than other groups. Nutritional variations also exist, such as lactose intolerance, which is common among Mexican, African, Asian, and Eastern European Jewish Americans.
- Social organization. This refers to the family unit and social group organizations, such as religions ones, with which patients and families may identify.
- Communication. Communication differences can present themselves in many ways. There are language differences, which can include verbal, non-verbal, and silent communication. Communication is important in all stages of the patient–therapist relationship. Clear and effective communication is important. When communication is not achieved the therapist can become frustrated and ineffective. Accurate assessment, diagnosis, and treatment are impossible. The patient can become hostile, belligerent, uncooperative, and withdrawn. If the patient does not speak the dominant language an interpreter should be employed.
- Space. "Territoriality is the term for the behavior and attitude people exhibit about an area they have claimed and defend or react emotionally about when others encroach on it" (Spector, 2000, p. 87). Different cultures attach different meanings to space. There is intimate space, which extends up to 1.5 feet; personal space, which extends from 1.5 to 4 feet; social space, which extends from 4 feet to 12 feet; and public space, which extends 12 feet and beyond.

- Time orientation. How cultures view the past, present, and future varies among groups. Cultures in the United States and Canada tend to be future-oriented and are therefore concerned with future long-range goals and preventative measures. These people like to make schedules, set appointments, and organize activities. Others are oriented to the present and may be late to appointments. Time orientation is important to consider when planning appointments and medication schedules.

## Health traditions

Health-tradition models use the concept of holistic health—including body, mind, and spirit—and explore how people maintain, protect, and prevent illness. The traditional ways of maintaining health are the active ways people go about their everyday lives attempting to stay well. These include engagement in activities of daily living, such as wearing proper clothing, eating and preparing traditional foods, and doing physical activity. Proper clothing can include headgear or head coverings. The foods that are eaten and how they are prepared contribute to the health of the individual. Traditional diets are followed, and food taboos and restrictions are obeyed (Spector, 2000).

Mental health is maintained through concentrating and using the mind for such activities as reading and doing crafts. Games, books, music, hobbies, and art are media that allow expression of the self and help maintain well-being.

Another key to maintaining health is the family closeness and support system, including prayer and celebrations. The strong identity with and connection to the family and community events are especially important.

The traditional practices used in the protection of health consist of (Spector, 2000, p. 103):

- The use of protective objects such as amulets—worn, carried, or hung in homes.
- The use of substances that are ingested in certain ways and amounts or eliminated, and substances worn or hung in the home.
- The practices of religion, such as the burning of candles, the rituals of redemption, and prayer. Some believe that illness and evil are prevented by strict adherence to religious codes, morals, and religious practices.

Health restoration in the physical sense can be accomplished by the use of remedies such as herbal teas, liniments, special foods and food combinations, massage, and other activities. Calling on a traditional faith healer, using teas or massage, and seeking family and community support can restore mental health. In the spiritual sense restoration can be accomplished through healing rituals: religious healing symbols, prayer, meditation, special prayers, and exorcism.

## Multicultural health practices

### Native American health practices

A basic principle of Native American culture is wholeness.

> All things are interrelated. This connectedness derives from the reality that everything is part of a single whole that is greater than the sum of its parts. Hence any given phenomenon can only be understood in terms of the wholeness out of which it comes.
>
> (Bopp, Bopp, Brown, & Lane, 1984)

The essence of a healthy life is gratitude, respect, and generosity. Wholeness is known by many names: *Kitchi Manitou* (the Great Mystery, Ojibway), *Wakan Tanka* (the Great Sacred or Great Spirit, Lakota), and *Acbadadea* (Maker of all things above, Crow). Health is understood in terms of wholeness. Thus there is always a spiritual component. According to Cohen (1998), "[h]ealth means restoring the body, mind, and spirit to balance and wholeness; the balance of life energy in the body; the balance of ethical, reasonable, and just behavior; balanced relations within family and community; and harmonious relationships with nature" (p. 47).

Spector (2000) stated that many Native Americans believe that if it is not an emergency they should be allowed to see their medicine man first and then receive medical care. The medicine man is a support person who encourages them to go to the emergency room of the hospital. The therapist must be aware of several factors concerning communication. First is the recognition of the importance of nonverbal communication. The therapist does more observing than providing information. This needs to be noted when evaluating the patient. This creates a problem when taking history. The patient expects the health provider to deduce the problem rather than do direct problem-solving. It is advisable to use declarative statements rather than questions. Also, it should be noted that Native Americans use a very low tone of voice. It is important to listen carefully, reduce distractions, and use direct eye contact. Do not say "Huh?" or "I beg your pardon?" Note-taking is taboo. Use memory skills rather than notes. Also, the patient's time orientation is not in the future, so they will likely be late to appointments, and it would be advisable to use walk-in clinics.

Methods of treatment vary among tribal nations. The most common are prayer, chanting, music, verbalism, laying on of hands, counseling, and ceremony. Prayers focus the patient's mind on the rehabilitation process. Cohen (1998) stated that among northern plains nations, the patient uses a wrap with a pinch of tobacco in a small pouch. This is called a "tobacco tie," and it is used in praying for health and divine help. The praying act itself is a healing process. Prayers are directed toward the highest good and closed with the expression "All My Relations" rather than the Christian "Amen." This statement is true to the philosophy that prayers are dedicated to the health, harmony, and balance of all, including the Great Spirit. Some prayers can be put to music. Most songs are accompanied by a regular drumbeat. The rhythmic beat of a drum is itself a healing agent. It creates an expanded sense of awareness of self and spirit. The Indian flute is an important instrument of self-healing, and using flute music in the occupational therapy clinic can help to empty the mind of worries and preoccupations during the treatment process.

Counseling is a major part of intervention. In conjunction with the healer, therapists need to emphasize health rather than pathology. Focus on the person's strengths rather than their weaknesses. Humor can also be used frequently. "The goal is not to return a person to an average or 'normal' state; instead, the goal is to help the patient actualize their fullest potential by discovering the gifts of Spirit" (Cohen, 1998, p. 53). The duration of therapy should be considered when treating an American Indian. A disease can have a slow or sudden onset, and so healing can occur quickly or over a long period of time. The intensity of therapy is considered more important than the duration. The healing process may not be a gradual process but what appears like a quantum leap. There is awareness that changes must be made that affect lifestyle and behavior. The therapist is wise to remember that after five centuries of "red–white" interaction, Native American healers are willing to participate in the health care community as long as patients are approached with respect and unpretentiously. It must be recognized that relieving suffering is a common concern, and no culture has a monopoly on healing. Healers do not follow written guidelines and are recognized in each tribe, and healing traditions are passed down from generation to generation through visions, stories, and dreams. A healer uses different healing techniques with each person (aidsinfonet.org, May 23, 2006).

### *Jewish health practices*

Judaism is based on the idea that human beings are a unity of mind, body, and soul. This is called a "biopsychic" entity. "If mind, body, and soul are one—and are created *b'tselem Elohim/in the image of God*—then it is wrong to abuse the body" (Robinson, 2000, p. 223). This concept is central to Jewish health practices. If mind, body, and soul are one, then there is an integral relationship between what is thought of as worship, ethics, and social action. "[T]o worship God one must perform not only the obligatory 'religious' rituals, one must also behave ethically towards other humans, and work for justice in the world" (Robinson, 2000, p. 223). To be a Jew is not only to celebrate the festivals and Shabbat, but to behave ethically in a business relationship, and to pursue the larger social good. It is much more than praying and showing up in the synagogue on all the holidays. To live a Jewish life also dictates holistic health practices when receiving care from a therapist. Jewish life is about a person's actions more than a person's beliefs. All Jews are not alike and they are categorized by denominations the way "they respond to the *halakhah's* ordinances for personal action and behavior" (Bickel & Jantz, 2002, p. 49). The *halakhah* are writings that reflect Judaism's own enlightenment and are common to orthodoxy. Each denomination reflects the believer's culture, customs, and traditions and is manifested in health practices (Diamant & Cooper, 1991). These denominations are:

*Orthodox Judaism.* This is the oldest and most conservative of the Jewish traditions. Orthodox Jews maintain that the Torah (first five books of the Bible) was authored by Moses and is relevant today. The Talmud explains the Torah's teachings. Many of the prohibitions affect daily living on the Sabbath. For example, the Torah prohibits the use of fire on the Sabbath. Today, this prohibition is applied to electricity; electricity is not used on the Sabbath. Any equipment or device that requires electricity such as an electric razor, telephone, or electric light would have to be used during the weekdays. Another activity that the Torah prohibits on the Sabbath is the use of an automobile. Motor vehicles are prohibited except for emergencies. It is important that Jews live in close proximity to their place of worship. Orthodox Jews keep kosher strictly; they observe dietary laws both at home and in the larger community, including hospitals and rehabilitation centers. Another activity of daily living is toileting. On the Sabbath patients will use pre-torn strips of toilet paper to avoid tearing. If the patient pre-tears toilet paper, leave the strips alone and do not throw them out. Orthodox Jewish patients will not fill out menus for the next day. Have them fill out menus through the weekend in advance. An orthodox Jew cannot directly ask the therapist to perform prohibited activities on the Sabbath, and the therapist may have to perform everyday activities that the patient would normally do. The Sabbath begins on Friday evening before sundown. It begins 18 minutes before sunset of Friday evening and continues for the next 25 hours, until at least three stars are visible after dark on Saturday night (Parr & Shapiro, 2000). These hours need to be observed by the therapist. If a home-health occupational therapist needs to make a visit, it is important to call before the Sabbath begins because it is possible that the family will not answer, and thus a wrong assumption could be made about whether the patient is at home.

Observant Jews do not mix dairy products with meat. There must be a six-hour space between eating meat and dairy products. These people keep two separate sets of pots and dishes, one for dairy products and the other for meats (Dresser, 2005). Kosher dietary laws are important to keep in mind when using food to teach orthodox Jews to feed themselves. The therapist should talk to the patient about their eating habits before using cooking as a means of therapy.

> Orthodox Jews wash their hands in a ritual manner before eating a meal that includes bread. Hand washing is not required if bread is not served. It involves rinsing each hand twice with water poured from a cup and reciting a blessing.
>
> (Parr & Shapiro, 2000, p. 35)

The reason for this ritual is that it purifies the hands because they are touching impure objects.

It is okay to serve frozen kosher meals. The meal should be served hot. If it is allowed to cool off, it can be reheated but must not be opened and then reheated.

The patient will not eat the food if it has been opened. Let the patient open it or open it in the presence of the patient. Any food served from the clinic should have a kosher certification. Kosher-certified food will have a symbol on the package. There are many symbols, so do not rely on the "K" symbol. Check with the patient's rabbi if the therapist not sure.

In regard to dress, the *yarmulka* (skullcap) is a head covering worn by men as a symbol of their religious commitment and can be made of many fabrics and in many colors. It is worn during prayer, meals, or religious services. A *talit* (shawl) is worn around the shoulders. It can be worn over the head during morning prayer. Sometimes a Jewish man will wear a *talit katan* under the clothing all day.

> This garment is rectangular and smaller than the talit. It has an oblong cutout in the middle for the head, and falls over the chest and back. Some men keep the four knotted fringes (zitzit) on each corner exposed at all times.
>
> (Parr & Shapiro, 2000, p. 32)

It is important when teaching activities of daily living to remember that the Torah teaches modesty and dignity of the human body and that it must be protected. Some older Jewish people dress in their European tradition. Some men will grow beards and long side locks.

To maintain the modesty and dignity of the patient, remember that orthodox Jews will not touch or shake hands with people of the opposite sex. Orthodox women will always cover their knees and elbows and wear clothing with high necklines, hemlines below the knee, and full-length sleeves. Married women may cover their hair with a scarf at all times. Most orthodox women are prohibited from wearing slacks because the Torah forbids women to dress like men.

Orthodox Jewish men in hospitals and nursing homes may prefer that touching, especially personal care, be provided by a male therapist. Some will not consent to being touched by any woman except their wife. If it is not possible for a male Jew to have a male therapist, be sensitive to their feelings. Tell the person that they will be treated professionally, with respect and dignity. Explain what is to be done and why it must be done. The same courtesy should be shown to a woman when a man is providing care.

*Conservative Judaism.* Conservative Jews accept the divine origin of the Torah's message but believe that the teachings can be adapted to modern life. Conservative Judaism emphasizes the human relationship to the creator. It maintains the prohibition of working on the Sabbath, but it relaxes the laws on travel. Some conservative Jews observe the dietary laws but allow themselves more freedom in public. Some permit women to participate in religious services.

*Reform Judaism.* Reform Judaism is the most liberal. Most North American Jews follow the reform tradition. A reform Jew (not *reformed* Jew) follows the ethical laws of Judaism, but few follow the dietary and clothing customs. They believe that the Torah was not divinely written, so interpretation is more liberal.

The emphasis is on the prophetic teachings of the Bible, social ethics, and activism. There is no prohibition against driving or using electricity. Women are integrated into the religious life and can participate in religious services. Women can even serve as rabbis and cantors (Parr & Shapiro, 2000).

*Smaller Jewish movements.* Other Jewish traditions are considered movements rather than denominations. These traditions are reconstructionist, humanistic, Zionist, and Hasidic. During the evaluation process the therapist needs to note these Jewish traditions. *Reconstructionists* are considered a radical group. They are committed to a Jewish life but do not adhere to any specific rituals or beliefs. However, they may participate in Sabbath or dietary observances. There is total equality of men and women. The *humanistic* movement is the newest, and it is a non-theistic approach that does not commit to any formal religion. Many humanistic Jews are agnostic. They celebrate the importance of the individual, the culture, and history of Judaism but do not pray to a deity. They may participate in the Jewish holidays and ceremonies (Parr & Shapiro, 2000). *Zionism* is a movement whose purpose is to establish a Jewish state in response to oppression and loss of identity. It is important to note that when delivering health care, helping a patient maintain their identity is paramount. Zionism is close to orthodoxy. *Hasidism* is a movement that began in the 18th century in Poland. The Hasidic ("pious") movement emphasizes joy and emotion as opposed to book-learning and intellectualism. It is another movement that is close to orthodoxy (Bickel & Jantz, 2002).

### Islamic health practices

Islam is the fastest-growing religion in the world. It was once thought of as a middle-eastern religion. Islam is in such regions as Europe (Bosnia); Africa (Sudan, Somalia, Nigeria, Egypt); Southeast Asia (Indonesia, Malaysia, Thailand, Philippines, China, India); and the Middle East. Worldwide there are approximately 1.5 billion Muslims. The majority of Arabs are Muslims. There are seven million Muslims in the United States. "There are more Muslim Americans than there are Episcopalians, more Muslims than members of the Presbyterian Church USA, and as many Muslims as there are Jews" (Eck, 2001, p. 2). It is very difficult to get precise religious data because Public Law 94-521 prohibits the census bureau from asking questions about religious affiliation; therefore, data are gather by private associations. It is wise to keep in mind that Muslims follow Islam and not all Arabs follow Islam. There are many different Islamic cultures, and there are many differences other than faith. Individual interpretations of religious and cultural ideals, together with health care realities, mean that there are no definitive or universal applications of Islamic health care practices and beliefs. However, there are some similarities in health care practices and beliefs (www3.baylor.edu, February 4, 2007).

As with other religions there are divisions within Islam. These include differences between fundamentalists and secularists and between Sunni and Shi'a. Islam reaches across cultures, and health practices may be influenced more by culture than by religion. The Sunni make up 87% of all Muslims, and the rest are Shi'ites. For the purposes of this book the distinction will not be addressed, for the dispute between them is internal. The division made in this book is between the mystics of Islam, called Sufis, and the remaining majority of the faith, who are equally good Muslims but are not mystics (Huston, 1991).

With a growing Muslim population in the United States, the chance of a Muslim coming to a health clinic is likely to increase. Knowing the culture and religion of a patient enhances communication and effective health care. Some of the concepts of Islam are identical to those of Judaism and Christianity and its forerunners: God, creation, the human self, and the Day of Judgment (Huston, 1991). Therefore, some health practices come from these religions.

> Muslims view illness and death with patience and prayers. They consider an illness as atonement for their sins. They consider death as a part of a journey to meet their Lord. However, they are strongly encouraged to seek treatment and care.
>
> (www.islam-use.com, February 4, 2007)

Arab culture and Islam emphasize maintaining good health, through personal hygiene practices and a healthy diet. Western medicine is held in high esteem, and Muslims will seek medical assistance. The patient and family will not wait long to receive professional help and will want to receive medication as soon as possible. They are happy to answer any questions; they will listen carefully to the health professional's advice, explanations, and warnings and will follow instructions carefully. However, once symptoms have subsided they are likely to discontinue treatment and not follow up with scheduled appointments.

An Arab patient seeking medical treatment expects to be relieved from pain after receiving medication on the first visit. It is therefore important that the patient be relieved from discomfort before leaving the clinic. Patients like to have therapists explain the reasons for treatment. Nurses are perceived as helpers. Occupational therapists are not perceived as helpers, and the patient will not take suggestions and advice from them. The physician needs to explain the occupational therapist's role to the patient. Arabs are not accustomed to the profession of social work. The role of the social worker needs to be explained to the patient when referring. However, the patient relies on family and friends to support and help (www.culturediversity.org, May 30, 2019; www.naffcclinics. org, May 30, 2019).

Generally, both male and female Arab patients, both adults and children, prefer to be seen by male therapists. It is common for a family member to be with the patient during treatment so that any questions about the patient's health can be given with accuracy. Some Arab cultures believe that only good news should be given to the patient about their disease. It is appropriate for the physician to report the seriousness of the illness to a selected family member.

In times of distress or illness, the Muslim finds the greatest solace and comfort in the remembrance of God. The severely ill person, who might be distracted by pain, appreciates a person who can read the Qur'an. It is appreciated if the therapist asks the nearest Islamic center to send someone to someone to read to the patient. Visiting the sick is a basic duty one Muslim has for another, and is not necessarily reserved for close friends and family. Therefore, the Muslim patient will have many visitors during their course of treatment during the day. To visit another Muslim friend or relative is a form of worship.

The Qur'an does not address the issues of sickness and physical health. There are religious obligations and customs associated with religion that affect health care practices. Athar (2007) provides the occupational therapist a can do list for their Muslim patients.

- Cleanliness is required; the mouth, hands, and feet are washed at least five times each day. In preparation for prayer the patient will clean any waste from their body, clothing, and area of prayer. The person washes their hands, forearms, mouth, nostrils, face (wiping the top of the head and ears), and finally the feet. Patients who are physically challenged may use a dry cleansing (called *tayammum*) in which they strike their hands on a hard surface and then brush their palms over their hands and face.
- Modesty is important, especially for those individuals who have sexual awareness. Men and women are expected to behave conservatively. It should be noted that women use a *hijab* to keep their hair covered in public, and some may cover everything but the eyes and hands. Health and personal care or assessments from different-gender persons usually are distressing to more conservative or less cosmopolitan Muslims. Complaints or responses to questions may be edited by the patient based on the gender of the therapist and/or the translator (www.imana.org, May 30, 2019).
- No pork or pork products, such as lard, are allowed, nor are alcoholic beverages or any food prepared with alcohol, such as some kinds of desserts. It is possible that hospitalized patients may restrict their diet to only food brought by the family, or they may eat only vegetarian or kosher foods. It is important to note that gelatin, as in Jell-O and marshmallows, is often derived from pig skins.
- Among Muslims from the Middle East, quick pain/symptom relief is expected.
- After death, non-Muslims should not touch the body.

IMANA guidelines suggest the following:

- Respect modesty and privacy.
- When teaching patients to feed themselves provide Muslim or kosher meals.
- Allow Muslims to pray if they can. Provide them the space and the time to pray. All attention is directed toward the worship of God. Do not interrupt. The patient will continue until he or she is finished. The Muslim prayer takes approximately 5 to 10 minutes to complete. Help Muslim patients determine which direction is east.

- Inform Muslim patients of their patient rights.
- Take the time to explain procedures and treatment methods.
- Allow their imam (spiritual healer) to visit them.
- Allow the family to bring food if there are no restrictions.
- Always assess female patients in the presence of another female.
- Identify Muslim patients with the word "Muslim" in the charts and medical records.
- Provide a same-sex health care professional when possible.
- Provide spiritual comfort. When ill or sick the Muslim finds the greatest solace and comfort in the remembrance of God. Reading the Qur'an comforts them. Notify the nearest Islamic center for assistance.

### Oriental health practices

Dresser (2005) discusses customs, religious, and ethnicities of various Asian practices. The rehabilitation clinic is foreign to the Chinese. The environment is strange because they are not accustomed to the sights and smells of the health clinic. This tends to isolate the individual from their people, which creates a language barrier and feeling of helplessness. Food is another barrier to the individual, as they may be unaccustomed to the food that is served in the clinic. The typical Chinese person rarely complains and talks about what bothers them. The only symptoms may be the untouched food tray and the silence. The danger is to assume that the withdrawing behavior is a sign of compliance and good behavior. These patients may be viewed as stoic if there is no awareness that there may be deep-seated problems. This may result in a great deal of suffering.

Dresser (2005) states that among those of Asian/Pacific Island origin there are cultural beliefs regarding mental health and illness. Mental illness is much ignored. Two points must be noted: (1) the importance placed on family in caring for the mentally ill, and (2) the tendency to identify mental illness in somatic terms. There is a tremendous amount of stigma attached to mental illness. Therefore mental illness is often identified late, and patients may come with a feeling of helplessness.

Traditional methods of health maintenance and protection include amulets to prevent evil spirits. These are yellow paper charms hung over doors, pasted on a curtain or wall, worn in the hair, or placed in a red bag and pinned on clothing. The paper is burned and mixed with tea and swallowed to ward off evil. Jade is viewed as a giver of children, health, immortality, wisdom, power, victory, growth, and food. Charms made of jade are worn to bring good health. Children wear jade charms to keep them safe, and adults wear them for purity and intelligence.

Health restoration includes physicians and health care professionals, but they are not permitted to touch a woman's body. Various methods are used for diagnosing. Acupuncture is an ancient practice of puncturing the body to cure disease or relieve pain. Specific points of the body, known as meridians, are pierced with needles. Acupuncture is based on the concept that certain (365) meridians extend internally throughout the body in a fixed network (nccih.hih.gov, May 30, 2019). Herbal remedies are widely practiced. In addition to herbs and plants the Chinese use other products with medicinal and healing properties. An individual may use herbal remedies in conjunction with Western medicine. It is important to note any use of herbs that might interact with traditional medicine, such as herbs used with sleeping pills.

Dresser (2005) discusses various Asian cultures and their table practices. Chinese, Japanese, Korean, and Vietnamese people generally use chopsticks of various lengths that can be made of either wood or metal. Japanese people drink soup by lifting it to the mouth, whereas Koreans and the Chinese use soup spoons. Koreans use spoons to eat rice, but the Chinese and Japanese do not. When setting the table or teaching people to eat, be aware that Cambodians, Laotians, and the Hmong to not use forks and rarely use spoons. Laotian and Hmong people will use their fingers when eating sticky rice. People from Asian countries rarely set knives on the table. Dresser (2005) stated that when eating with the fingers, the right hand is used because the left hand is considered unclean. After the individual is finished eating, the chopsticks are placed in a parallel position across the top of the plate or bowl, but never on the table, never crossed, and never upright.

### Buddhist health practices[1]

#### Brief overview of Buddhism

Rahula (1959) has recounted the life story of the Buddha. About 2,500 years ago, the Buddhist religion began in northern India. It was developed by a real person, Siddhartha of the Gautama family. He was of noble birth and, after observing the suffering of mankind, he set forth to seek a solution to alleviate this suffering. He eventually became enlightened via meditation and a spiritual practice. "Buddha" means the enlightened one. One who is enlightened is fully aware and self-actualized. As explained by Chodron (2001), anyone can become and be called Buddha by cleansing the mind of defilements and realizing one's full potential.

Chodron (2001) has stated that the essence of Buddhism is to avoid harming others and to help others as much as possible. Interestingly, Zimmer (1956) stated that Buddhism offered no mythology or creed to believe in, but was more of a method or process of healing. He saw the Buddha as a spiritual healer.

Although begun in India, Buddhism spread eastward to China, Korea, Japan, and, more recently, to North America. In 2001 in the United States, Buddhism was listed as the fifth-largest religious group with an estimated adult population of 1,082,000. From 1999 to 2001, Buddhism grew 170% (Kosmin, Mayer, & Keysar, 2001). In the author's experience, the main components of Buddhism are the study of and adherence to the teachings of the Buddha, meditation, and fellowship with followers of the spiritual path.

American Buddhists I have met may combine Buddhism with another spiritual practice such as Christianity or Judaism. In my opinion, this is because

Buddhism provides a philosophy of living and is a stress-reducing practice rather than worship of a deity. All in all, Buddhism is becoming a common choice of spirituality that therapists need to recognize.

According to Rahula (1959), a major element of Buddhist teachings is the Four Noble Truths, which are related to suffering due to unsatisfactory experiences. These truths are (1) the truth of suffering, (2) the cause of suffering, (3) the cessation of suffering, and (4) the path to cessation. This first truth is that life is suffering and pain. Suffering is viewed as mental and spiritual, and it is interpreted in the widest sense of the term. Buddhism looks realistically and objectively to a person's life situation and tries to alleviate the innate lack of permanence, perfection, and stability. Included in suffering is birth, old age, sickness, grief, distress, separation from loved ones, and all kinds of unpleasantness.

Only brief descriptions of the Second and Third Noble Truths are offered in this writing. The Second Noble Truth examines the causes of suffering. According to Rahula (1959), the main cause of suffering is thirst or craving. This includes selfish desire for wealth, power, and pleasure. The Third Noble truth is that emancipation from suffering is possible. One has to give up thirst or desire. The main focus of the explanation of Buddhism in this work is how to get rid of thirst or suffering, which is contained in the Fourth Noble Truth.

*Buddhist practice*

The practice of Buddhism concentrates on the Fourth Noble Truth, which is the Cessation of Suffering. As Rahula (1959) explained it, practice takes a Middle Path between extreme, painful asceticism and seeking pleasure for happiness. It consists of what is termed an Eightfold Noble Path. There are three main elements of the Path. The first is ethical conduct, which is universal love and compassion for all living creatures. The second is mental discipline, which consists of (1) adherence to thinking in a positive and wholesome manner; (2) attentiveness to the body, feelings, mind, ideas, concepts, and other things; and (3) concentration, which involves maintenance of feelings of joy and happiness. The third element of the Path is wisdom, emphasizing the intellectual side and qualities of the mind. The intellectual side needs to meld with the compassionate side in happiness (Rahula, 1959).

Smith and Novak (2003) assert that the Eightfold Path consists of steps forming a treatment. It is beyond the scope of this writing to describe all the steps in detail. This writer has chosen to describe below what was felt that are the two most important steps for therapists to know.

Based on the above description, there is contained in the Path an important tenet of occupational therapy, which is incorporating a view of man as a holistic being, and therefore attending to body, mind, and feelings. The interaction of mind and body is important to health. Another important component of the Path, described by Smith and Novak (2003), is right livelihood. This "calls for engaging in occupations that promote life instead of destroying it" (Smith & Novak,

p. 44). Doing affects Buddhist spiritual practice. The kinds of occupations that are helpful or harmful depend on the historical time period and cultural context.

In summary, this brief overview presents Buddhism as not so much a religious experience rooted in belief, worship, and ceremony, but more as a spiritual practice of self-awareness, purification, and total well-being. According to Wilcock (1998), health from an occupational perspective includes (1) absence of illness (which is a kind of suffering), (2) physical, mental, and social well-being, (3) doing that which is socially valued (related to ethical conduct and right livelihood), and (4) the tenet of increasing human capacities and potential (self-development and aim of the Path).

## Health and Buddhism

Ikeda (1988) has written about the Buddhist view of health. Ikeda wrote that

> health is not just a state of freedom from negative influences, but a state in which one can actively solve problems. Through Buddhist practice, one can preserve health. Moreover, health and sickness are viewed as one, thus tying the healthy to the sick. Illness is a very important part of health, because it gives the impetus to attain a higher level of being. It moves a person to become more compassionate and help other people. Illness should not be a state to worry about, but to use for compassionate helping of others. For example, when a therapist gets sick, this enables insight, compassion, and action to develop. Buddhist medicine views the disease as a reflection of the total body system, or as life itself, and seeks to cure it not only through medical treatment, but also through adjustments in the person's lifestyle and outlook.
>
> (p. 66)

From this statement, the parallels between occupational therapy and Buddhism are made clear. Both emphasize mind and body interaction as well as lifestyle as a complex mix of occupations.

## Occupational therapy and Buddhism

A common element in mental and physical disabilities is pain. Martin (1999) described Buddhist practitioners' handling of pain. As he described and many therapists have discovered, most patients try to run away from their pain by doing; for example, they may go to the movies, watch television, or engage in some other diversional activity. This approach has been a mainstay in occupational therapy for decades and may be effective for some clients. Some other clients may spend a lot of energy and time in fighting the pain. Martin went on to explain that attending to pain by meditating on it and discovering all its nuances may actually soften it. The therapist may be able to make the pain more bearable. Martin used his own experience with depression to explain how noticing pain began to enable him to respond to it and get back into life.

Lastly, how do occupational therapists approach persons who are Buddhists? Bien (2006) asserted that therapists have to practice in a mindful way to help Buddhist therapist and ourselves as well. What is a mindful way? Bien explained mindfulness as a keen awareness of calm presence. It is fully experiencing reality and accepting that reality. Bien, in his book *Mindful Therapy*, explained how therapy done mindfully helps patients. Bien described reflective listening, allowing silence, the use of metaphor and story, and other methods.

## Summary

The chapter first addressed culture and its role in transmitting religious beliefs. Religious beliefs are then translated into health practices. Culture is the sum of beliefs, practices, habits, likes, dislikes, norms, customs, and rituals that are learned from families during the socialization process. Six cultural phenomena that affect health care are common among groups; these are environment, biological variations, social organization, communication, space, and time orientation. There are health traditions based on holistic concepts—including body, mind, and spirit—and that explore how people maintain, protect, and prevent illness. The health practices of Native Americans, Jews, Muslims, Orientals, and Buddhists were reviewed in the context of occupational therapy. Successful work with a diverse population necessitates viewing spiritual practice as a two-way street. The therapist has to meet the patient on his or her "playing field." In the case of the Buddhist, it is a therapeutic relationship wrapped in compassion, acceptance, mindfulness, ethical conduct, and wisdom that may result in the lessening of suffering and thereby contribute to effective habilitation and rehabilitation. Buddhism is not a religion, as defined in the American lexicon, but it is a way of thinking, doing, and being that may enhance client-centered care for practitioners.

## Note

1 © 2007 Nancy J. Powell. PhD. OTR, FAOTA Permission to print this unpublished manuscript. Dr. Powell is Associate Professor and Chairperson of the Occupational Therapy Program in the College of Health Profession at Grand Valley State University, Grand Rapids, MI.

## References

Kosmin, B. A., Mayer, E., & Keysar, A. (2001). *American religious identification survey 2001*. Graduate Center of the City University of New York. www.gc.cuny.edu/cuny_gc/media/cuny-graduate-center/pdf/aris/aris-pdf-version.pdf.

Athar, S. (2007). *Information for health care providers when dealing with a Muslim patient*. Islamic Downers Grove, IL, Medical Association of North America. www.islam-usa.com.

Bickel, B., & Jantz, S. (2002). *World religions & cults 101*. Eugene, OR: Harvest House Publishers.

Bien, T. (2006). *Mindful therapy: A guide for therapists and helping professionals.* Boston: Wilson.

Chodron, T. (2001). *Buddhism for beginners.* Ithaca, NY: Snow Lion.

Cohen, K. (1998). Native American medicine. *Alternative Therapies, 4*(6), 46.

Diamant, A., & Cooper, H. (1991). *Living a Jewish life: Jewish traditions, customs, and values for today's families.* New York: Harper.

Dresser, N. (2005). *Multicultural manners: Essential rules of etiquette for the 21st century.* Hoboken, NJ: John Wiley & Sons.

Eck, D. (2001). *A new religious America.* New York: HarperCollins.

Bopp, J., Bopp, M., Brown, L., & Lane, P. Jr. (1984). *The sacred tree.* Lethbridge, Canada: Four Worlds Development Project.

Giger, J., & Davidhizar, R. (1995). *Transcultural nursing assessment and intervention* (2nd ed.). St. Louis, MO: Mosby.

Huston, S. (1991). *The world religions: Our great wisdom traditions.* New York: HarperCollins?

Ikeda, D. (1988). *Unlocking the mysteries of birth and death ... and everything in between* (2nd ed.). Santa Monica, CA: Middleway.

Krefting, L. (2003). The culture concept in the everyday practice of occupational and physical therapy. In R. P. Fleming Cottrell (Eds.), *Perspectives for occupation-based practice* (pp. 201–207). Bethesda, MD: AOTA Press.

Martin, P. (1999). *The zen path through depression.* San Francisco: Harper.

Parr, M., & Shapiro, A. (2000). *Jewish resource guide: A caregiver's reference to the Jewish culture, customs and traditions.* Oak Park, MI: Singlish Publication Society.

Rahula, W. (1959). *What the Buddha taught.* New York: Grove Press.

Robinson, G. (2000). *Essential Judaism: A complete guide to beliefs, customs, and rituals.* New York: Pocket Books.

Smith, H., & Novak, P. (2003). *Buddhism: A concise introduction.* San Francisco: Harper.

Spector, R. (2000). *Cultural diversity in health and illness* (5th ed.). Saddle River, NJ: Prentice Hall Health.

Wilcock, A. A. (1998). *An occupational perspective of health.* Thorofare, NJ: Slack.

Zimmer, H. (1956). *Philosophies of India.* New York: Meridian.

# 8    Concepts on spiritual assessment/s

**Chapter objectives**

1   Describe the difference between religion and spirituality.
2   Identify how spiritual crisis or distress can occur.
3   State the eight worldview dimensions that should be included in a spiritual dimension.
4   Describe two factors likely to facilitate a successful discussion of spiritual dimension.
5   Identify the purpose of taking a spiritual history.

The therapist must distinguish between religion and spirituality. According to Hodge (2001), "religion flows from spirituality and expresses an internal subjective reality, corporately, in particular institutionalized forms, rituals, beliefs, and practice" (p. 204). Spirituality is definitely a part of religion, but religion may not be a part of spirituality. Spirituality contains the domains of religion, but a person can be spiritual without following religious ideology. Hodge (2001) defined spirituality "as a relationship with God, or whatever is held to be the Ultimate (for example, a set of sacred texts for Buddhists), that fosters a sense of meaning, purpose, and mission in life" (p. 204). This relationship results in concepts such as altruism, love, or forgiveness, which, in turn, affect a person's relationship to the self, nature, others, and the Ultimate Being (Carroll, 1997; Sernabeikian, 1994).

Many clinical assessments are limited by their use of terms that are broad enough that *spirituality* can be substituted for the word *God*, because some people are offended by the use of the word *God*. Some examples of alternative words for God could be transcendent being, deity, and higher power. These assessments generally assume that the client is Christian and do not include other traditions. The therapist must take precautions to not use measures that are based on Christian ideology when assessing people that are not of the Christian faith.

## Differences between assessing spirituality and religion

It has been seen that clinical assessments' ability to capture a client's spirituality is often limited by the choice of wording. As stated in Chapter 1, spirituality can be described using words such as *higher consciousness, transcendence, self-reliance, love, faith, enlightenment, community, self-actualization, compassion, forgiveness, mysticism, a higher power, grace,* and a multitude of other qualities. Any of these words can be used to describe a personal meaning concerning human life. A method of defining a concept can be accomplished by defining what it is *not.* For example, spirituality is not the practice of a religion and is not bound by dogma. The concern is that spirituality is often associated with religion and must be distinct from religion. The occupational therapist needs to be careful and use words that are consistent with the client's faith tradition.

A loss of meaning is the greatest crisis a person might experience when faced with illness or disease. People are able to face great physical and emotional trauma, but they might be unable to bear the sense of meaninglessness. People can overcome pain, disease, or hardship, but when they believe they are no longer needed, that they can no longer contribute, and that their life adds up to no meaning, they are in spiritual crisis (Howard & Howard, 1997). Hay (1989) and Smucker (1996) agree. Anandarajah and Hight (2001) add to the discussion about spiritual distress and spiritual crises and distress. The authors wrote that:

> Spiritual distress and spiritual crises occur when individuals are unable to find sources of meaning, hope, love, peace, comfort, strength, and connection in life or when conflict occurs between their beliefs and what is happening in their life. This distress can have a detrimental effect on physical and mental health. Medical illness and impending death can often trigger spiritual distress in patients and family members.
>
> (p. 86)

When a client is in spiritual crisis as defined by Anandarajah and Hight (2001), it is appropriate for the occupational therapist to administer a spiritual assessment, to initiate discussion about spiritual needs, and to refer the client to appropriate spiritual leaders if necessary. *Spiritual crises* and *spiritual distress* are "used to describe a pervasive disruption in a person's spiritual life" (Hasselkus, 2002). Spiritual crisis is the opposite of spiritual health, spiritual well-being, and spiritual integrity.

## Spirituality and the evaluation process

In 2002, the American Occupational Therapy Association's (AOTA) Commission on Practice developed the *Occupational Therapy Practice Framework: Domain and Process* (AOTA, 2002, 2008) to describe the clinical evaluation process. The *Framework* includes the creation of an occupational therapy profile and states that this:

is a summary of a client's occupational history and experiences, pattern of daily living, interests, values, and needs. Developing the occupational profile provides the ... practitioner with an understanding of a client's perspective and background.

(AOTA, 2014, p. S13)

The context is that described as the "overarching" influence on the treatment process and includes the client's spiritual locus of control and well-being, personal beliefs, level of spiritual maturity, and religious traditions and values.

Harold Koenig (2004) suggested four questions therapists can use when gathering information from clients about their spiritual history:

1  Is the client drawing on religion or spirituality as a method of coping with his or her illness?
2  Does the client have a supporting spiritual community?
3  Are there spiritual questions of concern to the client?
4  Does the client hold spiritual beliefs that may affect his or her medical care?

Similarly, Gorsuch and Miller (1999) proposed that therapists integrate the following three questions into the clinical setting during therapy:

1  Do you currently practice your religion?
2  Do you believe in God or a higher power?
3  Are there certain practices that you engage in on a regular basis?

They suggested that to assess a sense of meaning, therapists might ask, "What is important to you, and what gives you meaning and purpose in life?" These questions are helpful as we consider a spiritual assessment

Richards and Bergin (1997, pp. 172–187) proposed five reasons why spiritual assessment is essential in a therapeutic relationship:

1  To understand clients' worldviews so the therapist can become more empathetic and sensitive.
2  To increase the therapist's understanding of how healthy or unhealthy a client's spiritual orientation is and to what extent it affects the presenting problem.
3  To see whether the beliefs and the community can be used as resources for the client's coping methods and growth.
4  To find out which spiritual interventions may be beneficial for the client.
5  To determine whether the client has unresolved spiritual issues.

They also proposed eight dimensions that should be included in spiritual assessment:

1   Metaphysical worldview
2   Religious affiliation or denomination
3   Religious problem-solving style (i.e. a *self-directing* style is a problem solving process that involves only the self; *deferring* is problem solving that is given to God; and *collaborating* involves others, such as medicine healers)
4   Spiritual identity and tradition
5   God image
6   Value and lifestyle congruence
7   Doctrinal knowledge (i.e. the client's knowledge of sacred texts of his or her faith)
8   Religious and spiritual health and maturity.

(Richards and Bergin, 1997, pp. 172–187)

Gathering data does not constitute an assessment in itself; the information must be interpreted, organized, integrated with theory, and made meaningful (Rauch, 1993). *Assessment* is defined as "the process of gathering, analyzing, and synthesizing salient data into a multidimensional formulation that provides the basis for action decision" (Hodge, 2001, p. 204).

Spiritual assessment can sometimes raise concerns. Therapists must try to keep a balance between using and developing clients' spiritual strengths and remaining focused on their treatment goals. Therapy should always be the primary focus. The therapist needs to avoid assuming the role of spiritual expert and refer the client to his or her own spiritual or religious healer (Hodge, 2001).

When practitioners have firmly held values, they risk imposing their own positions on clients. In this case, they should not conduct spiritual assessments with people who hold values different from theirs. Conversely, some people consider spirituality a private matter and may object to exploring this area in a rehabilitative setting. Others do not believe in a higher being, and the therapist should respect this. In short, therapists should never administer a spiritual assessment without obtaining consent. Before entering into a discussion about religious beliefs with their clients, therapists should keep in mind the following general recommendations for taking spiritual history:

- Spirituality is a potentially important component of every client's physical well-being and mental health.
- Address spirituality at each complete period of reassessment, and continue addressing it at follow-up. In client care, spirituality is an ongoing issue.
- Respect a client's privacy regarding his or her spiritual beliefs; do not impose one's own beliefs.
- Make referrals to chaplains, spiritual directors, or community resources, as appropriate.
- Therapists should be aware of their own beliefs as well as how their personality will affect the therapist/client encounter, and they should try to make that encounter a more humanistic one.

Anandarajah and Hight (2001) promoted to two factors that can increase the likelihood of a successful discussion of spiritual needs. The authors labeled the factors *spiritual self-understanding* and *self-care.* They asserted that the therapist must understand their own spiritual beliefs, values, and biases to remain client-centered and nonjudgmental when dealing with the client's spiritual concerns. This concept is compatible with the relationship-centered concept mentioned in Chapter 2, and it is especially relevant when the therapist's and client's beliefs differ. Anandarajah and Hight (2001) stated, "Spiritual self-care is integral to serving the multiple needs and demands of patients in the current health care system" (p. 6). Koenig (2004) suggested some barriers to obtaining spiritual histories, including lack of time on the part of the therapist, lack of training, discomfort with the subject, worries about imposing religious beliefs on clients, and lack of interest or awareness. Therefore, it is important that therapists first look at their spiritual self.

## Therapist and client spiritual history—FICA

Puchalski (2005) suggested a self-assessment that therapists can use when taking a personal spiritual history. Both the self-assessment and the spiritual history tool are referred to as the FICA, for the initial letters of the four key concepts.[1]

- **F: Faith or beliefs**
  Do I have a spiritual belief that helps me cope with stress? With illness? What gives my life meaning?
- **I: Importance**
  Is this belief important to me? Does it influence how I think about my health and illness? Does it influence my health care decisions?
- **C: Community**
  Do I belong in a spiritual community (church, temple, mosque) or other group? Am I happy there? Do I need to do more with the community? Do I need to search for another community? If I don't have a community, would it help me if I found one?
- **A: Address**
  What should be my action plan? What changes do I need to make? Are these spiritual practices I want to develop? Would it help for me to see a chaplain, spiritual director, or pastoral counselor?

## Spiritual history assessment (FICA)

Therapists can use the following suggested FICA questions to take a history of clients' spirituality.

- **F: Faith and belief**
  Do you consider yourself spiritual or religious? Do you have spiritual beliefs that help you cope with stress? If the patient responds, "No," the

therapist might ask, "What gives your life meaning?" Sometimes patients respond with answers such as family, career, or nature.

- **I: Importance**
  Is this belief important to me? Does it influence how I think about my health and illness? Does it influence my health care decisions?
- **C: Community**
  Do I belong to a spiritual community (church, temple, mosque or other group)? Am I happy there? Do I need to do more with the community? Do I need to search for another community? If I don't have a community, would it help me if I found one?
- **A: Address**
  What should my action plan be? What changes do I need to make? Are there spiritual practices I want to develop? Would it help for me to see a chaplain, spiritual director, or pastoral counselor?

## Spiritual crisis

Illness and disability raise fundamental questions about spiritual well-being: Why me? Why do I suffer? Does my suffering have meaning? Maugans (1997) developed a framework for taking a spiritual interview and answering these questions based on the concepts of suffering from Viktor Frankl's (1946/1984) work *Man's Search for Meaning*. Frankl (1946/1984) stated that physical discomfort and deprivation, no matter how extreme or brutal, do not cause suffering. The cause of suffering is the loss of meaning and purpose in life. The following is an assessment developed by Maugans (1997):

The Spiritual History examines the concepts of meaning and purpose:

### S—Spiritual belief system

- Do you have a spiritual life that is important to you?
- Do you have a formal religious affiliation?
- What is your clearest sense of the meaning of your life at this time?

### P—Personal spirituality

- When you are afraid or in pain, how do you find comfort?
- Describe the beliefs and practices of your religion that you personally accept.
- In what ways is your spirituality or religion meaningful to you in your daily life?

### I—Integration with spiritual community

- Do you belong to any religious or spiritual group?
- How do you participate in this group?
- In what ways is this group a source of support for you?

**R—Ritualized practices and restrictions**

- What lifestyle activities or practices does your religion encourage, discourage, or forbid?
- What meaning do these practices hold for you?
- To what extent do you follow these practices?

**I—Implications for medical care**

- Would you like to discuss religious or spiritual implications of health care?
- Are there specific elements of medical care that your beliefs/religion discourage/forbid?
- Are there any persons you would like us to include in your spiritual care planning?

**T—Terminal events planning**

- Are there any unresolved areas of your life at this point that you would like us to assist you with addressing?
- Are there practices or rituals you would like available in the hospital or home?
- For what in your life do you still feel gratitude even though you are in pain?

The therapist should keep in mind the following hints for conversations about suffering and faith:

- Let the client set the agenda; the therapist does not need to ask about fear unless the client opens the door to the subject.
- Do not underestimate the power of silence. Sometimes the best support is simply listening.
- People generally are not looking for advice, just someone to listen and affirm that their fear, anger, sadness are normal.

## Observational assessments

Spiritual assessments come in a variety of formats but generally assess the same concepts. They can range from long written inventories to brief verbal inquiries and various kinds of surveys. The following assessment is in the format of an interview.

### *Assessment of spiritual well-being: observational cues*

**1   Current situation**

a   What religious or spiritual practices are important to you?
b   In what ways are they important to you?
c   How does your practice involve a community of other persons? Tell me about that community. How do you experience it?

d    Are there ways in which your religious/spiritual beliefs and practices influence this situation—the presenting problem?

## 2    History

a    Was religion or spirituality important to your family of origin? How so?

b    What beliefs and practices were important to your parents or those who cared for you?

c    Was there a religious community in which you participated as a child? What was the nature of that participation?

d    Did you attend religious services as a child?

e    Did the intensity or frequency of your religious practice vary when you were growing up?

f    If so, what happened that led to those changes?

g    What was the influence of your parents' spirituality on you? On your siblings?

## 3    Spirituality in this event

a    Are there concerns you have about how our talking might affect your spirituality or spiritual development?

b    Do any people who care for you (spouse, parent, child, etc.) have any such concerns?

c    Do you have any hopes/wishes about how your spirituality might help you in this process?

## 4    Assessment issues

a    Spirituality may function positively, negatively, or benignly in a person's life. The sincerity of the belief or the intensity with which it is held is not a measure of its healthfulness.

b    What is the impact of this person's spirituality on [his or her] life?

1    Motivation: how is what [he or she] is doing in the current situation influenced by spirituality?

2    Impact on defenses and mysticism?

3    Resources for growth/development within the spiritual tradition/ community.

### *Spiritual assessment guidelines (friends spiritual assessment)*

Another assessment in the form of a questionnaire is the Spiritual Assessment Guidelines by Marcia A. Schnorr, from the Friends General Conference of the Religious Society of Friends (2005). This was designed to be used for persons of the Quaker faith.

## 1    Source of spiritual strength

a    Who or what is your source of spiritual strength?

b   If your source of spiritual strength is God, how do you describe God? What does God mean to you?

c   If your source of spiritual strength is someone or something other than God, how do you describe this source? What does this source mean to you?

d   What objects and/or activities that you could use to maintain your relationship with your source of spirituality?

e   Are there other objects and/or activities that you could use to improve your relationship with your source of spiritual strength?

## 2   Meaning and purpose

a   What do you believe is the meaning and purpose for your life?

b   What activities help you to accomplish your purpose in life?

c   What purpose, if any, do you believe is served by suffering?

d   What do you believe is the meaning of death?

## 3   Love and relatedness

a   What is (are) your most significant relationships?

b   How would you describe these relationships?

c   How do you perceive that you are loved by others?

d   What are your main support systems?

e   Do you have a significant relationship with God? If so, consider the following question: If not would you like to have a relationship with God? (If a relationship is desired, serve as a resource and/or make the appropriate referral.)

f   How has your relationship with God been a source of help or hindrance in your life?

g   How do you feel about your relationship with God?

h   Has your relationship with God changed over the years?

i   Does your relationship with God have any effect on the quality of your life?

j   What person(s) has (have) had the most influence in helping you establish (maintain) your relationship with God?

k   What activities do you do participate in to help you maintain (grow) in your relationship with God?

l   What effect, if any, does your relationship with God have on your relationship with others?

## 4   Forgiveness

a   Have you ever experienced feelings of guilt, anger, resentment, and/or bitterness?

b   If so, what effect do those feelings have on your sense of wellness?

c   How do you handle those feelings?

d   Is there a difference between your feelings when you are forgiving?

e   Do you have more difficulty in experiencing forgiveness from God, for-giveness from others, or forgiveness from yourself?

f   What resources do you use to help you accept forgiveness?

g   What other resources might be available for you to experience forgiveness?

h   What prompts you to forgive others?

## 5   Hope

a   Would you describe yourself as hopeful?

b   Is your "hope" realistic? Or is it more like "wishful thinking?"

c   Does your relationship with God have an effect on your sense of hopefulness?

d   Have you ever felt hopeless? If so, describe the situation.

e   What resources do you use to obtain (maintain) a sense of hope?

f   Are there other resources that you could use to obtain (maintain) a sense of hope?

## 6   Effects of illness

a   Would being sick (injured) make any difference in the perception you have of yourself and God?

b   In what way, if any, do you perceive that your relationship to God is related to your present state of disease or dis-ease?

c   What resources do you use to relieve any spiritual distress related to your disease or dis-ease?

d   What other resources, if any, could you use to relieve your spiritual distress?

## 7   Religious affiliation

a   Are you affiliated with a particular religion? If so, which one?

b   What was the main factor in your choice of religious affiliation?

c   Is there any part of your religious life that may be influencing your feel-ings of wellness (distress)? (The interviewer may need to make an objective appraisal after further interactions and observations.)

d   What individual(s) has (have) had the most influence on your present religious practice (or lack of religious practice)?

e   Has any religious experience had an influence (positive or negative) on your present religious attitudes and practices?

f   What Bible character (story) do you most identify with at the present time?

g   What activities are most meaningful to you in your present religious life?

h   Are there any religious activities that you find most meaningful? Would you like to resume these activities?

i   How would you describe your sense of religious well-being?

### Engleside Skilled Nursing and Rehabilitation Center Assessment Tool

Engleside's assessment is rooted in a theory of logo therapy developed by Viktor Frankl (1946 /1984), a Viennese psychiatrist who survived several World War II concentration camps. Frankl (1946/1984) stated that people can find meaning in the presence of suffering and can transcend the horrors of life. He believed that people search for meaning in life up until the moment of death. By using a spiritual assessment to gather information, therapists can develop a treatment plan based on the experiences a person most values and wishes to retain. This tool is used to assess the meaning of a higher power to the patient.

Part I of the assessment gives information about the client's "concept of a God or deity, religion practices and helping others" (p. 1). Part II of the assessment examines the client's sources of help and strength, relation between spiritual self and health and impending death. Some questions included in this section are as follows: What are your personal goals? Do you want to participate in or assist with religious services at the facility? Are there roles you had in your life before that now you cannot do? What has given your life meaning in the past? What gives your life meaning now?

*Part I: activities*

Concept of God

1 Is religion or a god important to you?
2 Is prayer helpful?
3 Does a god play a role in your life?

Customary routine: involvement pattern

1 Do you find strength in your religious faith?
2 Do you usually attend church, temple, synagogue, etc.?
3 Are there any religious practices that are important to you?

Religious practices

1 Has being sick made any difference in your religious practices or prayer?
2 What religious books/reading or songs are helpful to you?
3 Have you participated in/would you be interested in a religious study of your faith?

Helping others

1 Do you enjoy helping others?
2 In what ways have you helped others?

*Part II: social services*

Sources of hope and strength

1    Who is the most important person to you?
2    Are there roles you had in your life before that now you can no longer do?
3    If so, how do you feel about this?
4    What gives your life meaning now?
5    In what ways do others help you?
6    What helps you most when you feel afraid or need special help?
7    What is your source of strength or hope?

Goals

1    What are your personal goals?
2    Do you want to participate in and/or assist with religious services?

Relation between spirituality and health

1    What do you think is going to happen to you?
2    Has being sick made any difference in your feelings or beliefs about God or religion?
3    Is there anything particularly frightening or meaningful to you now?

When the assessment is completed, the results are incorporated into the occupational therapy treatment plan. For example, if a client reports that he or she prays five times a day, the therapist works with the staff to provide private time for prayer; this should be written into the care plan. Family members can be encouraged to record familiar prayers for playing. In addition, family prayers and music can be incorporated into times of devotion.

## HOPE assessment

Administering a spiritual assessment as part of the data-gathering process is a step toward incorporating spirituality into the delivery of health care. The HOPE concept is as follows:

H—the source of hope, strength, comfort, meaning, peace, love and connection
O—the role of organized religion for the patient
P—personal spirituality and practices
E—the effects on medical care and end-of-life decisions.

Anandarajah and Hight (2001) reported that

> Ninety-four percent of patients admitted to hospitals believe that spiritual health is important as physical health, seventy-seven percent believe that physicians should consider their patients' spiritual needs as part of their

medical care, and thirty-seven percent want their health care provider to discuss religious beliefs more.

(p. 81)

The authors noted that "Spiritual assessment is the process by which health care providers can identify a patient's spiritual needs pertaining to medical care" (p. 87).

The HOPE questions serve to introduce spiritual content into the interviewing process. The questions have not yet been validated by research, but they allow open-ended inquiry into the client's spiritual resources and concerns. In the interview process, a therapist can ask, "For some people, their religious or spiritual beliefs act as a source of comfort and strength in dealing with life's ups and downs; is this true for you?" If the answer is "yes," the assessment can proceed. If the answer is "no," the clinician can ask, "Was it ever important to you?" If the answer is "yes," the clinician can follow up by asking, "What changed?" This can lead to further inquiry, or the therapist can cease asking questions about spiritual matters. The following are sample questions for use in the HOPE assessment.

### *Examples of questions for the HOPE approach to spiritual assessment*

#### H:  Sources of hope, meaning, comfort, strength, peace, love and connection

1  We have been discussing your support systems. I was wondering, what is there in your life that gives you internal support?
2  What are your sources of hope, strength, comfort, and peace?
3  What do you hold on to at difficult times?
4  What sustains you and keeps you going?
5  For some people, their religious and spiritual beliefs act as a source of comfort in dealing with life's ups and downs; is this true for you?

   • If the answer is "yes," go on to **O** and **P** questions.
   • If the answer is "no," consider asking, "Was it ever?" If answer is "yes," ask; "What changed?"

#### O:  Organized religion

1  Do you consider yourself part of an organized religion?
2  How important is this to you?
3  What aspects of your religion are helpful and not so helpful to you?
4  Are you part of a religious or spiritual community?

#### P:  Personal spiritual practices

1  Do you have personal spiritual beliefs that are independent of organized religion?

2    Do you believe in God? What kind of relationship do you have with God?

3    What aspects of your spirituality or spiritual practices do you find most helpful to you personally (e.g., prayer, meditation, reading scripture, attending religious services)?

**E:    Effects on medical care and end of life issues**

1    Has being sick (or your current situation) affected your ability to do the things that usually help you spiritually, or affected your relationship with God?

2    As a doctor, is there anything that I can do to help you access the resources that usually help you?

3    Are you worried about any conflicts between your beliefs and your medical situation/care/decisions?

4    Would it be helpful for you to speak to a clinical chaplain/community spiritual leader?

5    Are there any specific practices or restrictions I should know about in providing your medical care (e.g., dietary restrictions, use of blood products)?

6    If the patient is dying: How do your beliefs affect the kind of medical care you would like me to provide over the next few days/weeks/months?

## The Multidimensional Spiritual/Religiousness measure

The Multidimensional Spiritual/Religiousness measure shows some quantitative research. It is comprehensive, lengthy, and complex and is included in Appendix B for the reader's convenience. A booklet of the Multidimensional Spiritual/ Religiousness measure can be obtained free from the Fetzer Institute website along with a literature review, psychometric data, and analysis. There is a presentation of how the assessment is administered and scored. The research that has been conducted shows a level of validity with other spiritual assessments. Most research was with various populations. The working group has stated that the results support the theoretical basis of the measure; it has the appropriate reliability and validity to facilitate further research that will "help us better understand the complex relationship of religion, spirituality, and health" (Fetzer Institute, 2007, p. 89).[2] The main constructs examined that are related to health care are: daily, spiritual experiences, meaning, values, beliefs, forgiveness, private religious practices, religious/spiritual history, commitment, organizational religiousness, and religious preference. The advantage of this assessment is that it has a short form and a long form and the entire assessment does not have to be administered to obtain results.

# Summary

This chapter discussed the difference between religion and spirituality and presented spiritual assessments; both self-assessments and spiritual histories. Such assessments generally take the form of interviews, questionnaires, and inventories. Most assessments included in this chapter are qualitative. There are no published articles to date that demonstrate the benefits of taking a spiritual history, although there is some indirect evidence in support of this practice. First, spiritual practices are a way that patients are able to cope with medical illness. Second, spiritual beliefs have been found to influence medical decisions. Third, the patient's faith community is a source of support and found to be associated with adherence to medical therapy. Fourth, patient satisfaction with the emotional aspects of care is high (Koenig, 2004). It is suggested that the most appropriate time to take a spiritual history is during the initial assessment and history taking. The purpose of the spiritual history is to learn how the client copes with illness, and the kind of support system available to the client. It is possible that spiritual needs are not important to the client and the client may not believe that spiritual matters are important. At this point the occupational therapist does not need to go further and ask questions. So it is important not to "force a spiritual history upon patients who are not religious, coercing patients to believe or practice in specific way, providing spiritual counsel to patients, and activity that is not patient-centered and arguing with patients over religious matters" (Koenig, 2004, p. 2881).

Spiritual assessments usually focus on health care and end-of-life issues (e.g., one of these was HOPE). Therapists should consider administering a spiritual assessment at the beginning of the evaluation process and again at reevaluation. They should also complete spiritual assessments themselves to ensure that their own values and spiritual ideas do not influence their client's decisions. Spiritual issues can be approached as an aspect of diversity and treated with the same respect as any other personal issue (Openshaw & Harr, 2005). Spirituality is embedded in the client's culture and is expressed through health care practices. The next chapter addresses the culture diversity that affect a client's spirituality related to health care.

# Active learning strategies

1  Identify three to five questions you could pose to a client during completion of an occupational profile to evaluate their spirituality. How does this differ from evaluating religion? How do these questions relate to FICA?
2  From the spiritual assessments presented within the chapter, which would be the easiest for you to administer? Which would be the most challenging? Why?

## Notes

1 Reprinted from *Spiritual assessment tool, innovations in end-of-life care* (p. xx) by C. Puchalski, 1999. Unpublished manuscript. Copyright 1999 by Christina Puchalski, MD, FACP, director, George Washington Institute for Spirituality and Health. Reprinted with permission from author.
2 Reprinted from *Multidimensional Measurement of Religious/Spirituality for Use in Health Research* by the Fetzer Institute and the National Institute on Aging Working Group, 2007, available at www.fetzer.org. Copyright 2007 by Lynn G. Underwood, professor of biomedical humanities and director, Center for Literature, Medicine and Biomedical Humanities, Hiram College.

## Web resources

Spiritual Assessment Tool: www.hpsm.org/documents/End_of_Life_Summit_FICA_References.pdf.
Spiritual Care in Emergency Medicine: www.med-ed.virginia.edu/courses/culture/PDF/marcuschapter007spiritualcarerevisedgc.pdf.
Spiritual & Cultural Sensitivity in Healthcare: www.healthcarechaplaincy.org/user images/Cultural_Spiritual_Sensitivity_Learning_%20Module%207-10-09.pdf.

## References

American Occupational Therapy Association (AOTA). (2002). Occupational therapy practice framework: Domain and process. *American Journal of Occupational Therapy, 56*, 609–639.
American Occupational Therapy Association (AOTA). (2008). Occupational therapy practice framework: Domain and process (2nd ed.). *American Journal of Occupational Therapy, 62*, 625–683.
American Occupational Therapy Association (AOTA). (2014). Occupational therapy practice framework: Domain and process (3rd ed.). *American Journal of Occupational Therapy, 68*, S13.
Anandarajah, G., & Hight, E. (2001). Spirituality and medical practice: Using the HOPE questions as a practical tool for spiritual assessment. *American Family Physician, 63*, 81–89.
Carroll, M. (1997). Spirituality and clinical social work: Implications of past and current perspectives. *Arete, 22*(1), 25–34.
Frankl, V. (1984). *Man's search for meaning.* New York: Washington Square Press. (Original work published 1946)
Gorsuch, R., & Miller, W. (1999). Assessing spirituality. In W. Miller (Ed.), *Integrating spirituality into treatment: Resources for practitioners* (p. 293). Washington, DC: American Psychological Association.
Hasselkus, B. (2002). *The meaning of everyday occupation.* Thorofare, NJ: Slack.
Hay, M. (1989). Principles in building spiritual assessments tools. *American Journal of Hospital Care, 6*, 25–31.
Hodge, D. (2001). Spiritual assessment: A review of major qualitative methods and a new framework for assessing spirituality. *Social Work, 46*(3), 203–213.
Howard, B., & Howard, J. (1997). Occupation as spiritual activity. *American Journal of Occupational Therapy, 51*, 181–185.

Koenig, H. (2004). Taking a spiritual history. *Journal of the American Medical Association, 291,* 2881.

Maugans, T. (1997). The SPIRITual history. *Archives of Family Medicine, 5,* 11–16.

Openshaw, L., & Harr, C. (2005). *Ethical issues in spiritual assessment.* Botsford, CT: North American Association of Christians in Social Work.

Puchalski, C. (2005). Spiritual assessment tool, innovations in end-of-life care. *Journal of Palliative Medicine, 3*(1), 131.

Rauch, J. B. (1993). *Assessment: A sourcebook for social work practice.* Milwaukee, WI: Families International.

Richards, S., & Bergin, A. (1997). *A spiritual strategy for counseling and psychotherapy.* Washington, DC: American Psychological Association.

Schnorr, M. A. (2005). *Spiritual assessment guidelines.* Friends General Conference of the Religious Society of Friends. Retrieved 2005 from www.Fgcquaker.org/library/ fastering meetings.

Sernabeikian, P. (1994). Our clients, ourselves: The spiritual perspective and social work practice. *Social Work, 39,* 178–183.

Smucker, C. (1996). A phenomenological description of the experiences of spiritual distress. *Nurses Diagnosis, 7,* 81–91.

# 9   Spirituality and ethics

This chapter discusses the integration of spirituality into the occupational therapy treatment process. It is not intended to present an exhaustive treatise on ethics. Ethical principles applied in the clinical setting have been addressed in several resources which readers are advised to consult (Slater, 2010, 2015; Purtilo & Doherty, 2011: Corey, Corey, & Callanan, 2011).

Incorporating spirituality into the treatment process can create ethical concerns for occupational therapists. Possible concerns might be imposing your own religious beliefs on the client, and/or addressing any possible spiritual crises the client may be experiencing. To avoid ethical difficulties such as dilemmas between a client's religious traditions and forms of treatment, therapists must assess their own spirituality and where they are on that journey; they need to understand how to incorporate their own spirituality into their practice. In addition, therapists need to understand how clients' values and religious beliefs influence clients' decision-making. Some people base their identity (also known as idiosyncratic things that make a person unique) on what is right and wrong, and some draw the spiritual aspect of life from meaning. For example, meaning has been linked to religiousness and a sense of purpose in life.

According to Nicholi (2002), C. S. Lewis compared the moral teachings of the ancient Egyptians, Babylonians, Hindus, Chinese, Greeks, and Romans and found that they were very much alike, especially in their emphasis on being unselfish. There is a universal law that people do not put themselves first that seems to exist; as Lewis (1952, p. 1) wrote; "selfishness has never been admired." This unselfishness is a form of altruism, which is included in the seven core values and attitudes of occupational therapy practice (Slater, 2015), and "guide the values, actions and attitudes of occupational therapy practitioners" (Slater, 2015, p. 162). Altruism is defined in the Preamble of the *Occupational Therapy Code of Ethics and Ethics Standards* as "demonstrating concern for the welfare of others" (Slater, 2015, p. 8).

Morality according to the *Occupational Therapy Code of Ethics* (Slater, 2015, p. 292) consists of "the normative structure of human practice, including specific rights and duties, rules and laws, ideals, virtues and vices. Morality may be culture-based or culture-driven." Ethics is a philosophical discipline and can be defined as the philosophical study of morality. Morality is often called "descriptive ethics" which describes existing moral views. Ethics can be subdivided into *normative ethics*, which attempts to determine what is right and what is wrong (usually expressed in "dos and don'ts"). The occupational therapy code of ethics is normative ethics. *Meta-ethics* is concerned with tasks such as analyzing moral judgments (e.g., genetics, human and animal experiments). Normative ethics tries to establish which moral views are justifiable and thus ought to be accepted. The difference between ethics and morality is that ethics is the study of behavioral values, deals with principles, and asks what is morally right or wrong. Morality has higher standard. The two can overlap. Being moral can be a synonym for being ethical but not the other way around. To further define normative ethics Mappes and DeGrazia (1996, p. 2) stated,

> In general normative ethics task is to advance and provide a reasoned justification of an overall theory of moral obligation, thereby establishing an ethical theory that provides a general answer to the question: What is morally right and what is morally wrong?

The task of applied normative ethics is to resolve specific moral dilemmas. The health care professions, such as occupational therapy, are concerned with this branch of ethics. Mappes and DeGrazia (1996) suggested the following criteria for use when applying an ethical theory:

- The implication of an ethical theory must be largely reconcilable with experiences of the moral life.
- An ethical theory must provide effective guidance where it is most needed, that is, in situations in which substantive moral considerations can be advanced on both sides of an issue.

(p. 5)

Thus, if an ethical theory can capture the underlying structures of moral thinking, then its implications are in accord with moral thinking

## Teleological and deontological ethical theories

Ethical theories are generally grouped into two categories: *teleological* and *deontological.* Mappes and DeGrazia (1996) explained that:

> any ethical theory that claims the rightness and the wrongness of human action is *exclusively* a function of the goodness and badness of the consequences resulting directly or indirectly from that action is a teleological theory ... A theory is deontological if it places limits on the *relevance* of teleological considerations. Thus, an ethical theory in which moral rightness and wrongness of human action is construed as totally independent of the goodness and badness of consequences would be only one kind, deontological theory.

(p. 6)

The best known teleological ethical theory is *utilitarianism*, which holds that if an action or behavior fits then it should be acceptable, and if it works for others then it should work in other situations (Pence, 1998, p. 11). Pence summed up the essence of utilitarianism as follows:

- Consequentialism: that is, consequences count, not motives or intentions.
- The maximization principle: the number of people affected by consequences matters; the more people who are affected, the more important the effect is.
- A theory of value (or of "good"): Good consequences are defined by pleasure (hedonic utilitarianism) or what people prefer (preference utilitarianism). A consequence being recognized as something that naturally or logically follows from an action or condition.
- A scope-of-morality premise: Each being's happiness counts as one and no more.

According to utilitarianism, right acts produce the greatest number of good consequences for the greatest number of beings.

Related to utilitarianism is another well-known teleological ethical theory, *ethical egoism*. Ethical egoism is defined when a person acts so as to promote his or her own self-interest, which is problematic, in that a person can take the ethical action that is flagrantly antisocial in nature (Mappes & DeGrazia, 1996). For example, a person may know that proselytizing in a medical facility is wrong but continues anyway, believing that he or she will not get caught. Ethical egoism incorrectly implies that proselytizing is morally the right thing to do.

Another problem with ethical egoism is that it is prone to inconsistency. Suppose an occupational therapist considers him- or herself obligated to promote his or her own religious beliefs. If the occupational therapy department encourages its employees to promote their religious beliefs, then the therapist is openly performing what he or she believes to be a public moral action. However, it is to the client's and employee's advantage that the department not act egoistically, and it follows that it would be immoral for the therapist to publicly advocate his or her beliefs (ethical egoism). Mappes and DeGrazia (1996) asserted that

> in reducing morality to considerations of personal prudence, it can be argued, ethical egoism destroys the very sense behind morality. Morality, it would seem, functions ... to restrict the pursuit of personal self-interest. It is not that morality prohibits the pursuit of personal self-interest; rather it functions to place limits on this pursuit.
>
> (p. 6)

## Kantian deontology

Immanuel Kant (1964, 1963) a German philosopher, rejected utilitarianism and developed a classic deontological theory. Whereas the basic principle of utilitarianism is that a person ought to act so as to produce the greatest balance of good over evil, considering everyone including himself or herself—the essence of Kant's ethics is respect for others. Kant drew his principle from the golden rule: "Do unto others as you would have them do unto you." Mappes and DeGrazia (1996) put it this way:

> It is strictly impermissible for person A to treat person B merely as a means because such treatment is incompatible with respect for B as a person. Notice that Kant does not claim that it is morally wrong for one person to use another as a means. His claim is that it is morally wrong for one person to use another as merely a means.
>
> (p. 18)

A therapist uses the data collected from the clinic as a means of conducting research or of gaining knowledge and skills. The therapist is using the client as a means of attaining information, but is also providing them with health care. Human subject review boards are formed at health institutions to safeguard this balance. Mappes and DeGrazia (1996) felt that "such human interactions ... based on an involuntary participation of respective parties, are quite compatible with a principle of respect for persons" (p. 18). This recognition of respect for others includes the acceptance of clients' rightful authority to conduct their life as they see fit, including their decisions to engage in any spiritual or religious activity.

Pence (1998, p. 8) summed up Kantian ethics by listing four elements:

1   Ethics is not a matter of consequences but of duty—why an act is done is more important that its good or bad results.
2   A right act has a maxim that is universalizable—an act is right if one can will all others to act on its "maxim" or rule. "Lie to keep getting out of keeping a promise," for example, cannot be so willed, because if everyone acted this way, promise-keeping would mean nothing.
3   A right act always treats other humans as ends in themselves, never as mere means.
4   People are only free when they act rationally—this is called *autonomy.*

## Prima facie duties

The philosopher W. D. Ross (1930) believed that neither Kant nor the utilitarian theories were helpful in conflicting situations. He proposed a deontological theory that provides defensible "cases of coincidence" that help people face situations in which one duty pulls from one direction and another duty pulls from another direction—i.e., conflicting moral dilemmas.

According to the *Reference Guide to the Occupational Therapy Code of Ethics & Ethics Standards* (Slater, 2015), a duty is "the idea that humans, although free to act otherwise, are bound to act in a particular way that is considered good or the norm" (p. 291). The Latin phrase *prima facie* literally means "at first glance." A prima facie duty is a conditional duty and can be overridden by other duties. Ross stated that people's duties emerge out of their "morally significant relations"; friend-to-friend, clergy-to-parishioner, and therapist-to-patient relationships. Ross further stated that people have "both a prima facie duty to keep promises and a prima facie duty to assist those who are in need" (p. 22). According to Ross, the duty to keep promises is usually more incumbent than the duty to assist those who are in need. Whenever the promise is trivial and the other action is a compelling choice, Ross would say that the latter choice should take precedence. He encouraged the person caught in an ethical dilemma to reflect on the circumstances when considering a given situation. Mappes and DeGrazia (1996) summarize Ross's categorization of prima facie duties as follows:

- Duties of fidelity—keeping promises, honoring contracts and agreements, and telling the truth—(as applied to occupational therapy, it also entails, honoring one's responsibilities as a therapist)
- Duties of reparation—wrongfully treating someone who creates the duty to rectify the wrong
- Duties of gratitude—being grateful for beneficial service provided by others
- Duties of beneficence—providing service to other people who can be made better
- Duties of non-maleficence—not injuring others
- Duties of justice—distributing benefits in accordance with personal merit and rectifying existing unjust patterns of distribution
- Duties of self-improvement—improving one's own condition (e.g., continuing education in the area of spirituality).

(pp. 22–23)

## Professional ethical issues

Ethical codes are necessary but not sufficient for the exercise of professional responsibility. Ethics in the health professions is regulated by both the laws and professional codes, which tend to be reactive rather than proactive; in that they are developed in response to events. Occupational therapists should act according to their conscience rather than a set of rules. Acting ethically is an inner quality, not something imposed by authority. In following their professional code, therapists are following "mandatory ethics." A higher level of ethical behavior is "aspirational ethics." Practitioners adhering to aspirational ethics go beyond what is required to be ethical. Mabe and Rollin (1986) listed the following limitations of professional ethical codes:

- Some issues cannot be handled by ethical code alone.
- Code enforcement may be difficult; courts or professional disciplinary boards may decide codes are not applicable.

- Codes often have internal contradictions and may conflict with other codes.
- The values of a practitioner may conflict with the code.
- Codes may conflict with institutional policies and practices.
- Codes tend to spring from past events rather than anticipate potential problems.

(pp. 294–297)

Similarly, Corey et al. (1988) stated:

Codes are not intended as a blueprint that would remove all need for use of judgment and ethical reasoning. Ethical codes tend to be conservative by nature. They are developed to protect the profession from outside regulation, and thus they reflect what most professionals can agree on, as opposed to reflecting ideal practice. Ethical standards cannot tell helpers what to do or why they should behave in a certain way. Final authority must rest with the therapist in determining what is right in a particular situation.

(p. 5)

The ethics of care pay attention to the affective components of moral life (i.e., moral behavior, moral values, moral character, moral reason, moral emotion, moral identity, meta-moral characteristics), with emphasis on empathy and concern for the needs of others. See Chapters 4–6 for a discussion of other characteristics of caring. A health care professional working within the spirit of ethics of care internalizes certain considerations (Mappes and DeGrazia, 1996, pp. 39–40):

- The individual needs, both physical and psychological, of the patient;
- How to respond in a caring, personalized manner to those needs;
- The likely impact of various options on the quality of the relationships among the involved persons, including the patient and professionals, but also other members of the healthcare team and any involved family members;
- How to respectfully attain and maintain the best possible relationships among those persons.

Nodding (2003) noted that conflict may arise between the perceived need of one person and the desire of another; between what the cared-for wants and what we see as his/her best interest; between the wants of the cared-for and the welfare of the persons yet unknown. We even find ourselves in conflict between two persons for whom we care and whose interests and beliefs are incompatible. Sometimes, the conflict cannot be resolved and must simply be lived (p. 55).

Gilligan (1982) researched moral developments to respond to the perspective of Kohlberg and Kramer (1996), whose findings suggested that men reach a higher level of moral maturity than women. Gilligan's (1982) research suggested just the opposite. Kohlberg and Kramer (1996) postulated three levels of moral maturity. The first level is the least mature, where children define right from wrong on the basis of authority. At the second level, people define right from wrong on the basis of loyalty to family. People achieve the third and most mature level when they come to rely on universal or abstract ethical principles, such as principles of justice and equality.

Gilligan's (1982) research showed that:

> The care perspective, the earliest level of moral development ... is one marked by a concern with caring only for oneself. At the second level, others become the focus of caring. At the third level, of moral development, the morally mature person achieves a balance between caring for others and caring for oneself.
>
> (p. 2)

Progression from stage to stage is dependent upon increasing one's understanding of human relationships and "maintain[ing] one's own integrity and care for one's self without neglecting others" (Andre & Velasquez, 1990, p. 2)

The inclusion of spiritual matters in the practice of occupational therapy, a health care profession, creates many ethical concerns for the therapist. Therapists can use the following guidelines to incorporate spirituality into the problem-solving process to avoid violating ethical principles (Openshaw & Harr, 2005).

1  Determine if there is an ethical dilemma.
2  Identify key values, principles, and knowledge central to the dilemma.
3  Prioritize relevant values and ethical principles.
4  Face any personal biases that could cloud your perspective.
5  Consult with colleagues about the dilemma as needed.
6  Develop an action plan consistent with the ethical values identified.
7  Implement the plan using the most appropriate practice skills and areas of competence.
8  Reflect on the outcome of the ethical decision-making process.

Occupational therapy recognizes religion and spirituality as important aspects of diversity and considers them in its ethical practices. For example, the preamble to the *Occupational Therapy Code of Ethics & Ethics Standards* (2010) states that

> Members of AOTA are committed to promoting inclusion, participation, safety, and well-being for all recipients in various stages of life, health, and illness and to empowering all beneficiaries of service to meet their occupational needs. Recipients of services may be individuals, groups, families, organizations, communities, or populations. Occupational therapy personnel have an ethical responsibility primarily to recipients of service and secondarily, to society.
>
> (p. S17)

Moreover, in its *Core Values and Attitudes of Occupational Therapy Practice*, AOTA (1993) stated, "We believe that we should respect all individuals, keeping in mind that they may have values, beliefs, or lifestyles that are different from our own" (p. 2). Another core value is that "we value human beings holistically, respecting the unique interaction of the mind, body, and physical and social environment" (AOTA, 1993 p. 3). AOTA's position paper *Occupational Therapy's Commitment to Nondiscrimination and Inclusion* states that "we value individuals and respect their culture, ethnicity, race, age, religion, gender, sexual orientation, and capacities, consistent with the principles defined and described in the Occupational Therapy Code of Ethics" (AOTA, 2005). These statements imply the requirement for an integrated pattern of behavior that respects the thoughts, communications, actions, customs, beliefs, values, and institutions of all racial, ethnic, religious, and social groups. They further suggest that the terms *diversity*, *social environment*, and *beliefs* include people of various cultures, religions, and sexual and gender orientations.

## The application of spirituality to AOTA principles of ethical standards

Many ethical principles are related to spirituality. Code and Ethics Standards Principles 1E and 1F address the importance of being competent in areas of practice and of critically examining emerging evidence to perform one's duties on the basis of current information. Even though this is about evidence-based practice, it can also apply to the therapist and using the true self and being aware of one's own spiritual journey, discussed in Chapter 1. It means to use the self to enhance success in therapy in connection with current practice treatment. Being aware of one's personal journey means examining the self in relation to medical practices. Accordingly, the therapist is responsible for self-analysis of his or her own religious beliefs and identification of what may cause a conflict between the client and therapist. If the client is asked to undergo medical treatment that is against his or her religious beliefs, the therapist should report the conflict to his or her supervisor. Similarly, if the occupational therapist cannot perform his or her duties because of his or her religious beliefs, he or she should be open to asking the occupational therapy supervisor to reassign the client to another therapist.

The principle further supports the core value of seeking to develop and understand one's own cultural values and beliefs as one way of appreciating the importance of multicultural identities. Education and the accumulation of knowledge are life-long processes for occupational therapists and are required for the therapists to maintain certification. Therapists can reach an understanding of diverse patients by gaining knowledge of cultural diversity (i.e., the existence of a multiplicity of sub-cultures and different value systems in a plural or multicultural society or other setting). Continuing education is essential in areas such as world religion and process theology.

According to Principle 1I, in the Code and Ethics Standards, "occupational therapy personnel shall refer to other providers when indicated by the needs of the client" (p. 9).

This principle includes referrals to clergy or other spiritual healers. It is important to be knowledgeable about services available in the community and broader society to make referrals for diverse patients (National Association of Social Workers, 2001). Clients may find support, both financial and relational, in religiously or spiritually oriented organizations. Faith groups such as churches, synagogues, or mosques should be identified. Failure to refer may show a negative bias against such groups:

- When one's own belief system prohibits involvement in the spiritual care of a client.
- When spiritual issues seem particularly significant in the client's suffering.
- When spiritual/religious beliefs seem of particular help and support for the client.
- When addressing the spiritual needs of a client exceeds the therapist's comfort.
- When the client needs specific community spiritual resources.
- When the client's family seems to be experiencing spiritual pain.

A therapist can refer at any time but should be cautious about putting the clients in contact with organizations or groups with which the therapist has no relationship.

Principle 2C of the Code and Ethics Standards directs occupational therapy personnel to "recognize and take appropriate action to remedy personal problems and limitations that might cause harm, to recipients of service, colleagues, students, research participants, or others" (p. 9). This statement includes the avoidance of evangelizing or proselytizing. In keeping with the concept of equality, therapists must respect all people, including those with differences in religious beliefs and lifestyle. *Respect* means prizing people because they are human (see discussion in Chapter 6).

Principle 3A of the Code and Ethics Standards states that "Practitioners have a duty to treat the client according to the client's desires within the bounds of accepted standards of care" (p. 10), and "also acknowledges a person's right to hold views, to make choices, and to take actions based on [his or her] values and beliefs" (p. 10). It is important to respect the holidays clients observe such as Ramadan, Christmas, Halloween, Holy Cross Day, or Passover. Holidays are often reflections or celebrations or religious events or rituals. Accordingly, therapists should understand the major world religions and be knowledgeable about the effects of cultural diversity. It is also worth mentioning differences in types of worship. Some religions hold their Sabbath on Saturday, some use rituals, and some include objects of worship.

Principle 3E of the Code and Ethics Standards gives the client the "right to refuse occupational therapy services, temporarily or permanently without negative consequences" (p. 10), including the right not to discuss his or her religious beliefs. The client may be a nonbeliever or an agnostic or may not think that religious beliefs have anything to do with health.

Principles 3G and H mandate that "Occupational therapy personnel shall ensure that confidentiality and the right to privacy are respected and maintained regarding all information obtained about recipients of service, students, research participants, colleagues or employees" (p. S21). This principle protects any communication about religion that the client considers privileged. With the current interest in spirituality, an increasing number of quantitative and qualitative studies have been conducted. Assessment development and results from spiritual assessments are used in a variety of settings and are kept in confidence, as are any other data.

Principle 4F of the Code and Ethics Standards applies to diversity.

> Occupational therapy personnel shall provide services that reflect an understanding of how occupational therapy service delivery can be affected by factors such as economic status, age, ethnicity, race, geography, disability, marital status, sexual orientation, gender, gender identity, religion, culture, and political affiliation.
>
> (p. S22)

It is important that therapists be aware that their own spiritual views may conflict with a client who has a different lifestyle and views. It is also important to recognize commonalities in a client's worldview, because those commonalities may cause the therapist to be biased in favor of results from assessment procedures or interventions. In addition, those commonalities (or lack thereof) could determine whether a therapist sees the client's religious beliefs to be a source of strength or pathology.

## Ethical application of spirituality to practice

This chapter discusses the application of spirituality to the practice of occupational therapy and ethical behavior in the clinical setting. The following set of universal ethics should guide clinicians' thinking as they interact with clients who are experiencing a spiritual crisis:

- Being human, being real: being honest, listening.
- Being present and listening: The emphasis is on being (with), not doing
- Including spiritual concerns in treatment planning.
- Respecting the client's belief system, regardless of one's own feelings about religion and spirituality.
- Providing access to spiritual resources by referring to spiritual healers, such as chaplains, parish priests, ministers, rabbis, and imams.
- Being a caring professional means encouraging clients and their family to give voice.

- Explore but do not probe, help people to feel heard, and be present.
- Avoid judging beliefs, practices, or emotional responses; refrain from proselytizing or imposing your own beliefs.
- Be aware of your beliefs and the impact they have on the health care process.
- Be careful if you and a client share the same religious traditions; beliefs and practices vary widely.
- Avoid discussion of doctrine, dogma, and complicated theological questions. The client usually does not want or need intellectual discussions. All he or she needs is comfort and reassurance.

  - When talking to clients avoid clichés such as "It is God's will" or "God never gives you more than you can bear." Do not use this language unless the client and family have used these phrases themselves.
  - Respect the client's and family's spiritual traditions and practices, as well as their privacy in this area.
  - Do not initiate participation in the client's religious observances. Let the family do the inviting.
  - Finally, follow the plan for spiritual care agreed upon by the client, family, and health team.

## Summary

The purpose of this chapter was to acquaint the occupational therapy therapist about the ethics of caring for patients in their treatment settings. Incorporating spirituality into the treatment setting is not an easy job. Suggestions were made about how spirituality could be integrated into the *Occupational Therapy Code of Ethics*. The specific principles were 1E, 1F 1I, 2C, 3A, 3C, 3G, and 4F. When establishing a relationship with a client who is receiving occupational therapy, the therapist should consider the client's spiritual practices, maintain a therapeutic relationship based on the client's spiritual needs, collaborate with the client's faith healer, respect the client's right not to share his or her religious tradition, participate in continuing education in areas of religious traditions and practices, and be current in research related to religious traditions.

Several ethical theories were reviewed. Each of them in essence states that the individual person, in this case a therapist, needs to determine what is right and what is wrong in a situation. It was recognized that what is right in one situation may be wrong in another. This depended on the set of moral issues. Culture determines what is morally right or wrong. Morality has a higher standard. The two can overlap. Being moral can be a synonym for being ethical but not the other way around. The author drew upon Kantian ethical theory and the concept of universality. Kant believed that reasonable people can use their minds and determine what is morally right without religion or external authority. Kantian theory was not helpful in conflicting ethical dilemmas which therapists frequently face. What was helpful was a concept called prima facie duties, which included duties of fidelity, reparation, gratitude, beneficence, non-maleficence, justice, and self-improvement. They are applied to the *Occupational Therapy Code of Ethics*. Beyond what is written, is aspirational ethics, which requires one to go beyond what is asked—beyond what is written in a code of ethics. The therapist uses judgment and reasoning to determine what is right and wrong. The ethics of caring is employed when written rules do not seem to apply during clinical practice. There is a selfless caring and a caring for others. There is a balance between oneself and others. This is the highest level of moral development. Therapists are faced with a dilemma when they are faced with equally attractive mutually exclusive alternatives. When there are no written rules that cover an ethical dilemma it is from personal moral characteristics from which to make hard moral decisions. A truly moral person is a person of moral discernment and uses virtual ethics to make ethical decisions. These characteristics are virtues that are derived from Judeo-Christianity and Islam. They are compassion, care, faith, and restraint (humility). Without compassion, health care ethics can become cold, meaningless, and very clinical. Compassion encompasses autonomy, justice, non-maleficence, and beneficence. Compassion is expressed in caring. And care is shaped by compassion. Being a caring person puts the patient first in a selfless environment. Faith/trust provides a powerful source of motivation to act selflessly. Humility relates to compassionate care and faith. Humility is a sense that the therapist does not know it all and needs to stay current in practice. There is recognition that there is more to know. These virtuous health care ethics are found in theistic traditions (Gill, 2006; Wogaman, 2009).

## References

American Occupational Therapy Association (AOTA). (1993). Core values and attitudes of occupational therapy practice. *American Journal of Occupational Therapy, 47*, 1085–1086.

American Occupational Therapy Association (AOTA). (2004). Occupational therapy's commitment to nondiscrimination and inclusion [position paper]. *American Journal of Occupational Therapy, 58*, 668.

American Occupational Therapy Association (AOTA). (2005). Occupational therapy code of ethics. *American Journal of Occupational Therapy, 59*, 639–642.

American Occupational Therapy Association (AOTA). (2008). *The reference manual of the official documents of the American occupational therapy association, Inc.* (13th ed., W. Schoen, Comp.). Bethesda, MD: Author.

American Occupational Therapy Association (AOTA). (2010). Occupation code of ethics and ethics standards. *American Journal of Occupational Therapy, 64*(6) (Suppl.), S17–26.

Andre, C., & Velasquez, M. (1990). *Issues in Ethics, 3*(1), 1–3.

Corey, G., Corey, M., & Callanan, P. (1988). *Issues and ethics in the helping professions.* Pacific Grove, CA: Brooks/Cole.

Corey, G., Corey, M., & Callanan, P. (2011). *Issues and ethics in the helping professions.* Pacific Grove, CA: Brooks/Cole Cengage Learning.

Gill, R. (2006). *Health care and Christian ethics.* Cambridge: Cambridge University Press.

Gilligan, C. (1982). *In a different voice: Psychological theory and women's development.* Cambridge, MA: Harvard University Press.

Kant, I. (1963). *On suicide (1755–1780): Lectures on ethics* (L. Enfield, Trans.). New York: Harper & Row.

Kant, I. (1964). *Groundwork of the metaphysic of morals* (H. J. Paton, Trans.). New York: Harper & Row.

Kohlberg, L., & Kramer, R. (1996), Continuities and discontinuities in childhood and adult moral development. *Human Development, 12*, 93–120.

Lewis, C. S. (1952). *Mere Christianity.* Westwood, NJ: Barbour & Company.

Mabe, A. R., & Rollin, S. A. (1986). The role of a code of ethical standards in counseling. *Journal of Counseling and Development, 64*(2), 294–297.

Mappes, T., & DeGrazia, D. (1996). *Biomedical ethics.* New York: McGraw-Hill.

Moyers, P. A., & Dale, L. M. (2007). *The guide to occupational therapy practice* (2nd ed.). Bethesda, MD: AOTA Press.

National Association of Social Workers. (2001). *NASW standards for cultural competence in social work practice.* Retrieved September 5, 2008, from www.socialworkers.org/sections/credentials/cultural_comp.asp.

Nicholi, A. (2002). *The question of God.* New York: Free Press.

Nodding, N. (2003). *Caring: A feminine approach to ethics and moral education.* Berkeley: University of California Press.

Openshaw, L., & Harr, C. (2005). *Ethical issues in spiritual assessment.* Botsford, CT: North American Association of Christians in Social Work.

Pence, G. (1998). *Classic cases in medical ethics.* New York: McGraw-Hill.

Purtilo, R., & Doherty, R. (2011). *Ethical dimensions in the health professions* (5th ed.). St. Louis, MO: Saunders/Elsevier.

Ross, W. D. (1930). *The right and the good.* Oxford: Clarendon Press.

Slater, D. (Ed.). (2010). *Reference guide to the occupational therapy code of ethics & ethics standards.* Bethesda, MD: American Occupational Therapy Association.

Slater, D. (Ed.). (2015). *Reference guide to the occupational therapy code of ethics & ethics standards.* Bethesda, MD: American Occupational Therapy Association.

Wogaman, J. (2009). *Moral dilemmas: An introduction to Christian ethics.* Louisville, KY: Westminster John Knox Press.

### *Related reading*

American Occupational Therapy Association (AOTA). (1998). Guidelines to the occupational therapy code of ethics. *American Journal of Occupational Therapy, 52,* 881–884.

# 10  Teaching spirituality in higher education

Since 1925, the Supreme Court has entertained growing numbers of cases having to do with religion and education. Justice Clark's often-quoted postscript to the majority decision in the 1960 *Schempp–Murray* case states "Nothing we have said here indicates that such study of the Bible or religion, when presented objectively as part of a secular program of education, may not be effected consistent with the First Amendment" (Engel, 1974, p. 41). Clark added that any question of religion in schools must be considered with great care and a feeling of sensitivity of others. Ordinarily, educators in federally funded schools do not have to think of legal opinions and public sentiments when developing content in a course, but religion is different from other activities and subjects in a curriculum. Nevertheless, higher education does include programs of study about religion. Universities are successful as well as legally liable because they are instruments of education and not vehicles for the practice of religion, but would also govern the teaching of spirituality in occupational therapy programs.

The academic study of religion is not the same as religious instruction, conversion, or spiritual direction. Religion was the last discipline to be academically accorded the neutral setting of research, debate, and free thinking that characterizes the university environment. The single greatest change that enabled religious studies to emerge as an academic discipline was the recognition that one can understand a religious position without adhering to it (Engel, 1974). Knowing about the tenets of a religion is quite different from believing in them. The academic study of religion depends on this distinction. At the most basic level, it is a descriptive discipline that gathers and disseminates accurate information about religious beliefs and practices (Gross, 1996). The course of study must be an interfaith approach that embraces all beliefs and religious traditions.

Spirituality is a concept within the study of religion; one can therefore teach it without teaching religious doctrine. The terms *religion* and *spirituality* should not be used interchangeably, because they are not the same (Egan & DeLaat, 1994). Spirituality, from an occupational therapy point of view is concerned with how a person perceives purpose and meaning in life; it is constructed through interconnectedness with others, the environment, and, for some, a higher power, which may be called God. Religiosity incorporates the practices, rituals, and rules of organized religion. Spirituality is definitely a part of religion, but the religion may not be a part of spirituality. Spirituality is recognized as an important concept in the study and practice of medicine. In occupational therapy, it is viewed as a part of the concept of holism. Any course in spirituality to be taught in an occupational therapy curriculum must begin with rationale.

## Rationale

When developing a rationale for a course of study in spirituality in occupational therapy, the instructor must keep four things in mind:

- The academic study of religion is a descriptive discipline that gathers and disseminates information about religious beliefs and practices. The course of study must have an interfaith and ecumenical approach that presents different worldviews. The major spiritual traditions as presented in Chapter 7, discussed a diversity of worldviews that the occupational therapist is liable to encounter. Depending on such factors as the demographics of the area which the course is being taught, it would be appropriate to include material that addresses traditions such as Mormonism, Islam, Judaism, Pentecostalism, Hinduism, Native American spirituality, and other traditions that might be common in the area.
- Spirituality is an important concept in the practice of medicine. Medical schools are now integrating spirituality into course content.
- Holism, a concept practiced by occupational therapists integrates spirituality and includes the concept of the therapeutic self. The therapeutic self, as part of the triad of holism—mind, body, and spirit—may be the vehicle through which one can engage in spiritual occupation.
- The therapist views spirituality within the scope of practice but lacks training.

## Course description

A sample course description for a course on spirituality in the practice of occupational therapy is as follows:

The purpose of this course is to provide the learner with the skills for developing a personal path for spiritual development. The content is designed to help the learner become aware of his or her spiritual path and the impact it has in occupational therapy treatment process. Journal work is introduced as a method of gaining insight into one's own stage of spirituality. Various definitions of spirituality are provided from the lay literature, health professional literature, occupational therapy literature, and theological literature. This is not a course in religion; however, spirituality as a religious concept in occupational therapy will be emphasized. The primary foci are the history of spirituality in occupational therapy, the theology of occupation, the therapeutic use of self, and the way in which spirituality fits into the treatment approach in occupational therapy treatment. These are the possible tools that therapists can use to assess a client's spiritual development.

## Course objectives

Learners will be able to:

- Identify the stages of spiritual development.
- Use a journal to gain insight into their own level of spiritual development.
- Express a personal definition of spirituality.
- Identify the role of spirituality in occupational therapy.
- Administer an assessment tool that measures spirituality.
- Discuss the history of spirituality in occupational therapy, including moral treatment and holism.
- Recognize the therapeutic use of self in occupational therapy treatment.
- Identify the domains of spirituality used in occupational therapy.
- Discuss the history of spirituality in occupational therapy.
- Identify spirituality concepts in the occupational therapy's professional official documents, including the *Occupational Therapy Code of Ethics* (Slater, 2015), *Standards of Practice for Occupational Therapy* (AOTA, 2005), the *Occupational Therapy Practice Framework* (AOTA, 2002, 2008, 2014), and official statements.
- Understand others' worldview—for example, Christianity, Judaism, Islam, atheism, agnosticism, Hinduism, and Buddhism.
- Understand spirituality as an occupation.

## Course activities

- Write a one page (typed, double-spaced, 250 word) personal definition of spirituality.
- Journal at least twice a week—one 250 word page.
- Write a page (typed, double-spaced, 250 word) paper answering the question "What role does spirituality have in occupational therapy?"
- Write a book report about religion different from one's own. This would help identify the differences between the student's own religious traditions and another's.
- Visit a church, synagogue, mosque, or other place of worship different from one's own, and write a five page reflection paper. This activity might include selecting a commonly encountered faith group whose value system differs substantially from their own and attempt to envision life through that particular worldview. By visiting a house of worship the student can note the difference in values.

- Administer a spiritual assessment. A common approach is to administer a spiritual history suggested in Chapter 8.
- A discussion of ethical issues concerning spirituality in practice.

These activities are designed to assist the student become competent by developing (Hodge, 2002, p. 92):

1   an empathetic understanding of a spiritually different worldview
2   an awareness of one's personal spiritual worldview and associated biases.

## Suggested lecture topics

A bibliography of resources is presented in Appendix D.

- Differences between religion and spirituality
- Definitions of spirituality
- Spirituality as an occupation
- Stages of spiritual development
- Moral treatment holism
- Therapeutic use of self
- Theology of occupation
- Theology of body and soul
- Spirituality in the occupational therapy documents (ethical code, standards of practice, etc.)
- Domains of spirituality
- The diversity of cultures and worldviews in occupational therapy.

## Suggested reading assignments

- Fetzer Institute. (1999). *Multidimensional measurement of religion/ spirituality for use in health research.* Kalamazoo, MI: Fetzer Institute.
- Fowler, J. (1981). *Stages of faith: The psychology of human development and the quest for meaning.* San Francisco: Harper-Collins.
- Hasselkus, B. (2002). *The meaning of everyday occupation.* Thorofare, NJ: Slack.
- Hemphill, B. (Ed.). (2007). *Assessments in occupational therapy mental health* (2nd ed.). Thorofare, NJ: Slack.
- Hemphill, B. (2008). *Spirituality for the common good: A theology of occupation.* Bethesda, MD: AOTA Press.
- McColl, M. (2003). *Spirituality and occupational therapy.* Ottawa, ON: Canadian Association of Occupational Therapists.

## Suggested resources

- American Occupational Therapy Association (AOTA). (2008). *The reference manual of the official documents of the American Occupational Therapy Association, Inc.* (13th ed.). Bethesda, MD: AOTA Press.
- Cottrell, F. (Ed.). (2005). *Perspectives for occupation based practice* (2nd ed.). Bethesda: AOTA Press (Chapters 24, 33, 35; pp. 204, 352–355).
- Kasar, J., & Clark, N. (2000). *Developing professional behavior.* Thorofare, NJ: Slack.
- Kornblau, B., & Starling, S. (2000). *Ethics in rehabilitation: A clinical perspective.* Thorofare, NJ: Slack.
- Kronenberg, F., Algado, S., & Pollard, N. (Eds.). (2005). *Occupational therapy without borders: Learning from the spirit of survivors.* London: Elsevier.
- Labovitz, D. (2003). *Ordinary miracles: True stories about overcoming obstacles and surviving catastrophes.* Thorofare, NJ: Slack.

## Classroom norms

Palmer (1999) stated,

> if you are in the room, your *values* are in there too—and if you do not believe that, you have not been paying attention. Students are quite adept at "psyching out" what their teachers believe. That is how students survive. When professors ... think they can mask who they are, they delude themselves and make the situation less trustworthy for others, contributing to the sense of danger that leads people to withhold self-investment.
>
> (p. 48)

The teacher's own spiritual journey is one of self-examination and growth. An active and intentional engagement in the journey of faith is respectful and includes open dialogue with the students.

The classroom must have norms so that participants can engage in a discussion of inquiry. Some leaders call these norms *boundary markers,* and some call them *discussion policies,* but they are rules that keep the group and each student focused. The purpose of these norms is to enhance understanding. For this to happen, an atmosphere of safety and respect must be created. The following are suggested possible norms:

- This is a course about spirituality, not religion. You will not need to bring your Bibles or any other sacred book.
- Each person is asked listen to others for the purpose of understanding.
- Each person has a right to and a responsibility for his or her own feelings, thoughts, and beliefs, and a right to discover what the disagreements are in the discussion/s.

- All religious traditions are to be respected. Everyone has a right to his or her own beliefs. There will be no proselytizing or preaching.
- Party politics are not permitted. Social justice issues may be permitted.
- Speak in the "I." You speak of how you believe, not how someone else ought to believe. Do not be dogmatic.
- What is said here stays here.
- Each person will suspend judgment. Avoid criticism or judgment of another person's feelings or point of view. Each student is asked to refrain from labeling any person as representing a group or position.
- Discussions are not arguments or debates. The classroom is for sharing ideas.
- Each person can express his or her theology. Disagreements are to be discussed in a civil manner.
- No one is to speak as though he or she has the "truth."
- We are students and teachers to each other. This is a laboratory for learning.
- Do not interrupt and make sure only one person is speaking at a time.

Each rule is designed to help create a caring atmosphere in which the goal is to learn about others, including the teacher. Each person is at some stage of spiritual development. To learn about the self and one's relationship to the universe is a worthwhile adventure. This course or something like it will meet the core component of the holistic endeavor in the therapeutic setting.

To introduce worldviews to students and to get into a frame of mind for class, instructors can begin each class with meditative music. Such music is often played on flutes, strings, or other non-vocal instruments. Students may be encouraged to bring a creative item to share with the class, perhaps a poem or reading from any tradition that expresses the student's spirituality. Each class begins and ends with a reading.

## Summary

This chapter has described a course that can be taught at a federally funded university at the college level, yet maintain the principle of separation of church and state. It encourages students to understand other worldviews and to examine their own spiritual journey. The objectives and class activities are designed to give students the means for integrating spirituality into the treatment setting. To develop a deeper, more personal understanding of other worldviews assignments should provide the opportunity to reflect on their experiences. It is critically important that resources continue to be developed that can equip occupational therapy students to practice spirituality in an ethically consistent manner. The student should be encouraged to develop a knowledge base about spiritual traditions that they are likely to encounter in the treatment setting. The information provided in the course curriculum is a beginning to lay the groundwork for spiritually competent practice. Topics in a course in spirituality should include:

1  Ethics and values
2  A review of literature on spirituality
3  Spiritual demographics of the region
4  An overview of the nation's major spiritual traditions
5  Assessment of spiritual strengths
6  Rights of spiritual believers
7  Assignment suggestions.

## References

Abington School District v. Schempp, 374 U.S. 203 (1963).

American Occupational Therapy Association (AOTA). (2002). Occupational therapy practice framework: Domain and process. *American Journal of Occupational Therapy, 56,* 609–639.

American Occupational Therapy Association (AOTA). (2005). Standards of practice for occupational therapy. *American Journal of Occupational Therapy, 59,* 663–665.

American Occupational Therapy Association (AOTA). (2008). Occupational therapy practice framework: Domain and process (2nd ed.). *American Journal of Occupational Therapy, 62,* 625–683.

American Occupational Therapy Association (AOTA). (2014). Occupational therapy practice framework: Domain and process. *American Journal of Occupational Therapy, 68,* s1–s48.

American Occupational Therapy Association (AOTA). (2015). Occupational therapy code of ethics. *American Journal of Occupational Therapy, 59,* 639–642.

Egan, M., & DeLaat, M. (1994). Considering spirituality in occupational therapy practice. *Canadian Journal of Occupational Therapy, 61*(2), 95–101.

Engel, D. (1974). Religion, education and the law. In D. E. Engel (Ed.), *Religion in public education* (pp. 41–51). New York: Paulist Press.

Gross, R. (1996). *Feminism and religion.* Boston: Beacon Press.

Hodge, D. (2002). Equipping social workers to address spirituality in practice settings: A model curriculum. *Advances in Social Work, 3*(2), 85–103.

Palmer, P. (1999). *The courage to teach: Exploring the inner landscape of a teacher's life.* San Francisco: Jossey-Bass.

# Appendix A

## References of affirmations

These resources can be used in the occupational therapy clinic or classroom. They are meant to be secular and not to advocate any specific faith tradition. These are what the author has found useful. Many similar resources can be obtained from a bookstore.

Brussat, M., & Brussat, F. (1996). *Spiritual literacy.* New York: Simon & Schuster.

Canfield, J., & Hansen, M. (1996). *A 3rd serving of chicken soup for the soul.* Deerfield Beach, FL: Health Communications.

Dreher, D. (1990). *The Tao of inner peace.* New York: Harper Perennial.

Fanning, P. (1994). *Visualization for change.* Oakland, CA: New Harbinger Publications.

Hanh, T. (1991). *Peace is every step.* New York: Bantam Books.

Haskell, B. (1994). *Journey beyond words: A companion to the workbook of the course.* Marina del Rey, CA: DeVorss.

Levine, S. (1991). *Guided meditations, explorations and healing.* New York: Anchor Books.

Naparstek, B. (1994). *Staying well with guided imagery.* New York: Warner Books.

Ryan, M. J. (1999). *Attitudes of gratitude: How to give and receive joy every day of your life.* New York: MJF Books.

Williamson, M. (1994). *Illuminata: A return to prayer.* New York: Berkley Publishing Group.

# Appendix B

## Multidimensional measurement of religiousness/spirituality for use in health research

*Table B.1* NIA/Fetzer short form, domains and instrument—GSS* results

| Domain | Testable relevance to health | 1998 GSS item wording |
|---|---|---|
| Affiliation | Denomination-specific proscriptions for lifestyle risk factors: alcohol, diet, smoking | What is your religious preference? Is it Protestant, Catholic, Jewish, some other religion, or no religion? |
| | | (If Protestant, what specific denomination is that?) |
| History | Life-changing experience fostering behavior change | Did you ever have a religious or spiritual experience that changed your life? |
| | Exposure to psychophysical religious/spiritual states | |
| Public practices | Exposure to psychophysical religious/spiritual states | How often do you attend religious services? |
| | Conformity to risk-reducing behaviors | How often do you take part in the activities or organizations of a church or place of worship other than attending services? |
| | Exposure to social networks and sources of support | |
| Private practices | Exposure to psychophysical religious/spiritual states | How often do you pray privately in places other than at church or synagogue? |
| | | Within your religious or spiritual tradition, how often do you meditate? |
| | | How often have you read the Bible in the last year? |

*continued*

*Table B.1* Continued

| Domain | Testable relevance to health | 1998 GSS item wording |
|---|---|---|
| Support | Access to instrumental assistance and expression of caring | If you were ill, how much would the people in your congregation help you out? |
| | Reduction of stress through resolution of conflict | If you had a problem or were faced with a difficult situation, how much comfort would the people in your congregation be willing to give you? |
| | Encouragement of compliance with medical treatments | How often do the people in your congregation make too many demands on you? |
| | Reduction of health risk behaviors | How often are the people in your congregation critical of you and the things you do? |
| | Access to medical care and health information through referral networks | |
| Coping | Reduction of negative impact of stressful life events | Think about how you try to understand and deal with major problems in your life. To what extent is each of the following involved in the way you cope: |
| | | I think about how my life is part of a larger spiritual force. |
| | | I work together with God as partners. |
| | | I look to God for strength, support, guidance. |
| | | I feel that God is punishing me for my sins or lack of spirituality. |
| | | I wonder whether God has abandoned me. |
| | | I try to make sense of the situation and decide what to do without relying on God. |
| Beliefs and values | Opportunities for social comparison promote personal well-being | I believe in a God who watches over me. |
| | | I feel a deep sense of responsibility for reducing pain and suffering in the world. |
| | Reduction of stress through provision of hope | Do you believe there is life after death? |
| | | I try hard to carry my religious beliefs into all my other dealings in life. |

*Table B.1* Continued

| Domain | Testable relevance to health | 1998 GSS item wording |
|---|---|---|
| Commitment | Enhancement of well-being through concern for others | During the last year, how much money did you and other family members in your household contribute to each of the following: |
| | | Other religious organizations, programs, causes? |
| | | Nonreligious charities, organizations, causes? |
| | | Were any of your contributions involved in the arts, culture, or humanities? |
| Forgiveness | Reduction of stress through resolution of conflict | Because of my religious or spiritual beliefs: |
| | | I have forgiven myself for things that I have done wrong. |
| | | I have forgiven those who hurt me. |
| | | I know that God forgives me. |
| Spiritual experience | Exposure to psychophysical religious/spiritual states | The following questions deal with possible spiritual experiences. To what extent can you say you experience the following: |
| | | I feel God's presence. |
| | | I find strength and comfort in my religion. |
| | | I feel deep inner peace or harmony. |
| | | I desire to be closer to or in union with God. |
| | | I feel God's love for me, directly or through others. |
| | | I am spiritually touched by the beauty of creation. |
| Religious intensity | Indicator of feelings of self-worth | To what extent do you consider yourself a religious person? |
| | | To what extent do you consider yourself a spiritual person? |

Source: Reprinted from *Multidimensional measurement of religious/spirituality for use in health research* (p. xx), by the Fetzer Institute and the National Institute on Aging (NIA) Working Group, 2007, available at www.fetzer.org. Copyright 2007 Lynn G. Underwood, professor of biomedical humanities, director of the Center for Literature, Medicine and Biomedical Humanities, Hiram College.

Notes
* 1998 General Social Survey, National Opinion Research Center, University of Chicago.
** R = respondent.

# Appendix C
## Spirituality in health care practice

Barnum, B. S. (1996). *Spirituality in nursing: From traditional to new age.* New York: Springer. The author explores the roots of spirituality in nursing as well as spirituality in relation to nursing theory (and theorists), healing, psychology, and ethics. She examines spirituality in light of an emerging paradigm that recognizes expanded consciousness as another way of apprehending "reality." Interesting reference lists at the end of each chapter contain books and articles from a variety of traditions (Christian, New Age, etc.). (Health Science Center (HSC) library—WY86 B263s 1996)

Boutell, K. A. (1990). Nurses' assessment of patients' spirituality: Continuing education implications. *Journal of Continuing Education in Nursing, 21*(4), 172–176. In a random survey, 238 Oklahoma nurses (of 817 solicited) returned usable questionnaires regarding the extent of their own spiritual assessment of their patients. The majority of these nurses "assessed their patients' spiritual needs from a moderate to considerable extent," with such factors as nurse specialty and time of day affecting the degree of assessment.

Burkhardt, M. A. (1989). Spirituality: An analysis of the concept. *Holistic Nursing Practice, 3*(3), 69–77. The author contrasts spirituality and religiosity, notes how researchers have studied the concepts, lists descriptive characteristics that emerge from the literature, and provides a definition of *spiriting* ("the unfolding of mystery through harmonious interconnectedness that springs from inner strength"). She notes the importance of "being with" the client and of listening for indications that the client has significant relationships and experiences of connection.

Carson, V. (1980). Meeting the needs of hospitalized psychiatric patients. *Perspectives in Psychiatric Care, 18*(1), 17–20. The author describes the experience and benefits of starting a prayer group in a unit of chronic psychiatric patients.

Cobb, M., & Robshaw, V. (Eds.). (1998). *The spiritual challenge of health care.* London: Harcourt Brace. Various authors address such topics as spiritual care, the meaning of spirituality in illness, faith, and spiritual values in a secular age. Pamela Reed presents an interesting multiparadigm model of spirituality. (HSC library—WM61 S753 1998)

Daaleman, T., & Nease, D. (1994). Patient attitudes regarding physician inquiry into spiritual and religious issues. *Journal of Family Practice, 39*, 564–568. Of 75 respondents in a convenience sample from a university-based clinic in Kansas, 64% indicated that they prayed daily. There was an association between (a) frequency of religious service attendance and (b) desire for physicians to inquire into patients' religious and personal faith and belief that physicians should make pastoral referrals. The authors referred to other studies indicating low levels of physician referrals to clergy at times of patient distress. Eighty-four percent of the study participants were Christian. The authors do not compare the sample with patients who refused to participate in the study, and partially completed surveys are included in the data set.

Dossey, L. (1999). Do religion and spirituality matter in health? A response to the recent article in *The Lancet. Alternative Therapies, 5*(3), 16–18. Dossey comments on Sloan, Bagiella, and Powell (1999; see below).

Eisenberg, D., Kessler, R., Foster, C., Norlock, F., Calkins, D., & Delbanco, T. (1993). Unconventional medicine in the United States. *New England Journal of Medicine, 328*, 246–252. In this hallmark study, 34% of 1539 randomly selected participants (participating in telephone interviews) reported having used at least one "unconventional therapy" in the past year. Seventy-two percent of these participants had not informed their doctor of the use. Twenty-five percent reported using prayer, which was second only to exercise as the most frequently used unconventional therapy.

Ellis, C. (1986). Course prepares nurses to meet patients' spiritual needs. *Health Progress, 67*(3), 7677. Ellis presents a brief discussion of a staff-development course on spiritual care that was formulated at St. Joseph Hospital in Houston, Texas, in 1985.

Emblen, J., & Halstead, L. (1993). Spiritual needs and interventions: Comparing the views of patients, nurses, and chaplains. *Clinical Nurse Specialist, 7*(40), 175–182. In this qualitative study, nurses, a convenience sample of surgical patients, and chaplains were asked to define *spiritual needs*, identify interventions, and note who they felt should attend to patients' spiritual needs. In order of frequency, talking, offering prayer, reading scripture, being present, and making referrals were noted as appropriate spiritual interventions.

Farran, C. J., Fitchett, G., Quiring-Emblen, C. J., & Burk, J. R. (1989). Development of a model for spiritual assessment and intervention. *Journal of Religion and Health, 28*(3), 185–194. The authors propose a multidisciplinary model for spiritual assessment and intervention. They define *spiritual dimension* in terms of a functional definition centered on meaning making, and they explore theoretical, developmental, and practical components of the spiritual dimension.

Flaskerud, J. H., & Rush, C. E. (1989). AIDS and traditional health beliefs and practices of Black women. *Nursing Research, 38*, 210–215. Using a focus group format followed by unstructured interviews of particularly knowledgeable participants, the authors explore the traditional health beliefs and practices of 22 low-income Black women in the Los Angeles area. In relating these to participants' beliefs concerning AIDS, the authors note supernatural as well as natural causes of the disease and found that prayer was viewed as a remedy and associated with healing. The article offers a good contrast of health care consumer and provider views of health and illness.

Highfield, M. (1992). Spiritual health of oncology patients: Nurse and patient perspectives. *Cancer Nursing, 15*(1), 1–8. In this descriptive, cross-sectional survey, the authors found no correlation between patients' self-assessed spiritual health and nurses' assessed health of these patients for 21 nurse–patient pairs.

Highfield, M., & Cason, C. (1983). Spiritual needs of patients: Are they recognized? *Cancer Nursing, 6*, 187–192. In this descriptive study, 35 nurses who worked with oncology patients responded to a questionnaire designed to assess their ability to recognize spiritual health in their clients. The authors conclude that the nurses had "limited ability" in this area.

King, D., & Bushwick, B. (1994). Beliefs and attitudes of hospital inpatients about faith healing and prayer. *Journal of Family Practice, 39*, 349–352. In this cross-sectional survey of hospital patients, 77% of the respondents said physicians should consider the spiritual needs of their patients, 48% wanted their physicians to pray with them, and

37% wanted more frequent discussions of religious beliefs with their physicians. Sixty-eight percent indicated that their physicians had never discussed religious beliefs with them.

King, D. E., Sobal, J., & DeForge, B. R (1988). Family practice patients' experiences and beliefs in faith healing. *Journal of Family Practice, 27,* 505–508. From a cross-sectional survey of 207 patients in a rural North Carolina family practice clinic, authors noted that 21% of the patients had attended a faith-healing service and 21% either had been healed or knew of someone who had been healed. Additionally, 58% of the respondents considered faith healers to be "quacks," whereas 29% believed that faith healers could help some people. The majority of respondents were female and Baptist.

King, D. E., Sobal, J., Haggerty, J., Dent, M., & Patton, D. (1992). Experiences and atti-tudes about faith healing among family physicians. *Journal of Family Practice, 32,* 158–162. Questionnaires were sent to a random sample of physicians in seven states. Of 594 respondents, 83% rarely or only sometimes discussed religion with their patients, although 93% agreed or strongly agreed that physicians should consider their patients' spiritual needs. Twenty-three percent of the physicians believed that some people could be healed by faith healers, and 16% had actually attended a faith-healing service.

McGlone, M. (1990). Healing the spirit. *Holistic Nurse Practitioner, 4*(4), 77–84. The author contrasts the terms *cure* and *heal* and notes how the quality of relationship differs in interactions leading to each. She notes that illness can actually be a cure for "time famine," allowing people to focus on spiritual concerns. She also briefly dis-cusses prayer and meditation, spiritual healing, and therapeutic touch.

McGuire, M. B. (1988). *Ritual healing in suburban America.* New Brunswick, NJ: Rutgers University Press. In this extensive study, researchers attended 255 group meet-ings and conducted 356 personal interviews in one New Jersey county to document local "alternative-healing" beliefs and practices. Models for conceptualizing illness and healing are described for Christian, metaphysical, Eastern meditation, and psychic healing groups. Adherents of many different alternative healing practices had views of health and illness that were "radically different" from those assumed by the dominant medical model. Many practitioners of prayer did not share basic assumptions regarding health and illness that are taken for granted by much of the health care community. Persons who practiced prayer often had very different conceptualizations of what needed to be healed and how that could happen.

McSherry, W., & Draper, P. (1998). The debates emerging from the literature surround-ing the concept of spirituality as applied to nursing. *Journal of Advanced Nursing, 27,* 683–691. The authors explore three debates emerging in nursing literature related to the concept of spirituality. These debates center on deriving a conceptual and theoret-ical view of spirituality that will be functional for the profession; reclaiming the spir-itual heritage of nursing in a milieu dominated by science, technology, and secularism; and viewing spirituality from a truly holistic perspective (whereby it is not reduced to one of several parts of our being but is understood to be impinging on, infiltrating, and penetrating "all areas of our life in a subtle way establishing meaning and purpose"). This insightful article examines some of the subtler aspects of the quest to understand spirituality within the health care arena. It includes a useful reference list with many citations related to spiritual care.

Marwick, C. (1997). Should physicians prescribe prayer for health? Spiritual aspects of well-being considered. *Journal of the American Medical Association, 273,* 1561–1562. The article reports on a meeting of the National Institute for Healthcare Research (attended by such researchers as Koenig, Levin, and Larson) at which the role of prayer and religion in maintaining health was discussed and future research needs were outlined.

Maugans, T., & Wadland, W. (1991). Religion and family medicine: A survey of physicians and patients. *Journal of Family Practice, 32,* 210–212. To investigate the role of religion in family practice medicine, the authors surveyed both physicians and patients. Physicians were less religious than were patients. Forty percent of patients were open to physician inquiry regarding religious issues, but actual physician inquiry was reported to be infrequent by both patients and physicians. In both groups, the majority of respondents acknowledged the utility of prayer and the existence of God.

Nagai-Jacobson, M., & Burkhardt, M. (1989). Spirituality: Cornerstone of holistic nursing practice. *Holistic Nurse Practitioner, 3*(3), 18–26. This article is an exploration of spirituality, including concepts such as attending to what one knows, interconnectedness, listening with one's being, connections with the sacred, and presence and silence.

Newman, M. (1989). The spirit of nursing. *Holistic Nurse Practitioner, 3*(3), 1–6. Newman discusses spirituality in relation to "pattern recognition" and "sensing into one's own field." For her, the nurse's task is to facilitate the "insight into his or her own pattern" (facilitated by a shared consciousness or connection).

Newshan, G. (1998). Transcending the physical: Spiritual aspects of pain in patients with HIV and/or cancer. *Journal of Advanced Nursing, 28,* 1236–1241. Spirituality is conceptualized to consist of hope, meaning, love, and relatedness in this article, which explores spiritual tools (including presence) the nurse may employ in the care of patients with pain.

Novack, D. H., Epstein, R, M., & Paulsen, R. H. (1999). Toward creating physician-healers: Fostering medical students' self-awareness, personal growth, and well-being. *Academic Medicine, 74,* 516–520. The authors discuss how programs designed specifically to foster self-awareness, personal growth, and well-being in medical students should result in physicians who are truly able to bring about healing as they use themselves as diagnostic and therapeutic instruments.

O'Brien, M. E. (1999). *Spirituality in nursing: Standing on holy ground.* Sudbury, MA: Jones & Bartlett. The history of nursing is traced through the Christian tradition, and spirituality is related to nursing roles in terms of caring, healing, and the provision of spiritual resources. Spiritual needs of the acutely ill, the chronically ill, children and families, older adults, the dying, and the grieving are specifically discussed. Reference lists contain many Christian-oriented books and papers.

Oyama, O., & Koenig, H. G. (1998). Religious beliefs and practices in family medicine. *Archives of Family Medicine, 7,* 431–435. The results of this survey indicate physicians to be less likely than their patients to have religious affiliations, pray privately, or hold intrinsic religious attitudes. Additionally, the more religious patients were, the more likely they were to want to know the physician's religious views and want the physician to pray with them.

Piles, C. (1990). Providing spiritual care. *Nurse Educator, 15*(1), 36–41. Of 176 nurses who responded to a survey (carried out across several diverse regions of the United States), 96.5% believed that holistic care involves spiritual care, but 65.9% felt inadequately prepared to perform such care. Knowledge and time deficits were noted as obstacles to providing care. The author includes a discussion of the difference between spiritual and psychosocial care.

Roush, W. (1997). Herbert Benson: Mind-body maverick pushes the envelope. *Science, 276,* 357–359. The author relates a brief history of Herbert Benson, a physician and researcher known for his work in mind–body medicine, the "relaxation response" and hypertension, and the belief that faith can be a powerful force in healing. Both supporters and detractors of Benson's work are noted, as are Benson's plans to replicate the Byrd study.

Sloan, R. P., Bagiella, E., & Powell, T. (1999). Religion, spirituality, and medicine. *Lancet, 353*, 664–667. In light of a growing interest in the interface of health and spirituality in the medical community, the authors examine empirical evidence and explore ethical issues related to physician involvement in this type of "nonmedical agenda."

Soderstrom, K., & Martinson, I. (1987). Patients' spiritual coping strategies: A study of nurse and patient perspectives. *Oncology Nursing Forum, 14*(2), 41–46. Among 25 oncology patients, prayer was noted as the most frequently used spiritual coping strategy, although the majority of patients used a variety of spiritual coping methods. Almost half of the patients used nurses as spiritual resources. Lack of time was noted by 76% of the nurses surveyed as detracting from their ability to incorporate spiritual assessments in nursing practice.

Stuart, E., Deckro, J., & Mandel, C. (1989). Spirituality in health and healing: A clinical program. *Holistic Nurse Practitioner, 3*(3), 35–46. The authors present a very interesting application of Herbert Benson's relaxation response within the clinical setting of a hypertension group program. This is a practical application of a mind–body–spirit approach.

Taylor, P., & Ferszt, G. (1990). Spiritual healing. *Holistic Nurse Practitioner, 4*(4), 32–38. The authors discuss such concepts as touch, accompaniment, and prayer in relation to healing and death.

Wells, B. (1999). Revival: Duke renews the ancient conversation between religion and medicine. *Duke Medical Perspectives, 19*(1), 30–37. New programs are being developed at Duke University as a result of a growing discussion between the schools of divinity and medicine. The Institute on Care at the End of Life, a parish nursing program, and a forum for health care providers to discuss spiritual issues grew out of this discussion. The history of religion and health, research on the effects of religion on health, and current trends linking the association of the two disciplines are briefly discussed. This article has no reference list.

Widerquest, J. G. (1991). Another view on spiritual care. *Nurse Educator, 16*(2), 5, 7. In responding to another article on spiritual care, this author speaks of the overlapping of spiritual and psychosocial needs and contrasts such terms as *religious* and *spiritual* as well as *curing* and *healing.*

# Appendix D
## List of potential instruments

On the basis of a review of 74 articles, I found 30 potential instruments for consideration. These are divided into four groups of scales that measure (1) quality of life, (2) attitudes, (3) religiousness, and (4) spirituality.

### *Quality of life*

Nine of these instruments are quality-of-life measures, which are mostly functional. Some have two or three questions related to spirituality. For the most part, however, they are functional assessments and therefore are not described in depth here:

- McGill Quality of Life Questionnaire (Cohen, Mount, Strobel, & Bui, 1995): Three of 20 questions are relevant to spirituality.
- Missoula-VITAS Quality of Life Index (Byock, 1995).
- McMaster Health Index Questionnaire (Chambers, Macdonald, Tugwell, Buchanan, & Kraag, 1982): Three questions of 24 are spiritual.
- MacAdam and Smith's (1987) index of quality of life: a section on spirituality in an index designed for the terminally ill.
- QL Index, HIRC-QL, Uniscale QL (Morris, Suissa, Sherwood, Wright, & Greer, 1986), administered as part of the National Hospice Study.
- Ferrans and Powers's (1985) Quality of Life Index: Four of 34 questions are relevant to spirituality.
- The Hospice Index (McMillan & Mahon, 1994): Three of 26 questions are relevant to spirituality.

### *Attitude indexes*

- Death Attitude Profile (Gesser, Wong, & Reker, 1987): a 21-item self-administered questionnaire for use with a general population.
- Life Attitude Profile (Reker & Peacock, 1981): a 36-item multidimensional profile developed and tested in a college population and more recently in hospitalized patients and outpatients. This is an excellent instrument for assessing spiritual needs but may need to be modified for a terminally ill population.

- McCanse Readiness for Death Instrument (McCanse, 1995): a 28-item structured interview questionnaire tested and verified in a terminally ill population. Four conceptual categories are included: withdrawal from internal and external environment, decreased social interaction, increased death acceptance behaviors, and increased admission of readiness to die.
- Templer's Death Anxiety Scale (Aday, 1984): a 15-item true–false structured interview questionnaire tested in a college-age population.
- Purpose in Life Test (Crumbaugh & Maholick, 1964): a 20-item attitude scale with emphasis on the need for purpose and meaning in life, used with patients with acute leukemia in the later stages of their disease. The measure was developed to test the concepts of logotherapy developed by Viktor Frankl.
- The Seeking of Noetic Goals Test (Crumbaugh, 1977): a 20-item scale that assesses the respondent's motivation to find additional meaning in his or her life.

### *Religiousness*

- Religious Coping Scale (Pargament et al., 1990): a 50-item scale with religious and spiritual as well as nonreligious, more psychological coping activities tested in a Christian church population. The authors draw some conclusions as to what types of religious coping mechanisms are helpful in difficult situations.
- Religious Orientation Measure (Allport & Ross, 1967): a 20-item self-administered questionnaire measuring the extrinsic (religion as a means to self-serving ends) and intrinsic (religion as an end in itself) dimensions of respondents. This is an extremely well-tested and widely used scale used to assess religiousness in many populations.
- Quest Scale (Batson & Schoenrade, 1991a, 1991b): a 12-item self-administered questionnaire introducing a third dimension to religiousness in addition to intrinsic and extrinsic—the quest dimension. Questions relate to life's meaning, the meaning of death, and of others. This measure was tested with a college-aged population and has been used with the general population but not specifically with hospital populations.
- The Religiousness Scale (Strayhorn, Weidman, & Larson, 1990): a 12-item self-administered scale tested and verified in families of Head Start children and subsequently used in the general population, including hospitalized patients and outpatients. This scale is good for determining the nature of people's religion: their commitment, their level of participation in their religion, and their relationship with God.
- Religious Coping (Koenig et al., 1992): a three-item index given by interview; each item measures how much the patient relied on religion to help manage emotional stress associated with an illness. The measure was tested in a Veterans Administration population of geriatric men and has been used in studies on depression.

*Spirituality*

- Spiritual Well-Being Scale (SWB; Paloutzian & Ellison, 1982): a 20-item self-administered scale with two dimensions: religious and existential. The measure was tested in a college population.
- Death Transcendence Scale (Hood & Morris, 1983; VandeCreek, Nye, & Herth, 1994): a 25-item self-administered scale based on the premise that "death is transcended through identification with phenomena more enduring than oneself." This scale has been tested in a diverse adult sample, including the hospital setting.
- Meaning in Life (ML) Scale (Warner & Williams, 1987): a 15-item scale administered by interview, tested in a facility for the chronically and terminally ill. The intent is for the patient to report his or her assessment of the worth of his or her remaining life.
- Herth Hope Index (HHI; VandeCreek et al., 1994): a 12-item interview containing three dimensions: temporality and future, positive readiness and expectance, and interconnectedness. The measure was tested in community members and in hospital patients and their family members.
- Index of Core Spiritual Experiences (Kass, Friedman, Leserman, Zuttermeister, & Benson, 1991): an 18-item interview scale used for spiritual assessment in the general population as well as with hospital patients.
- Spiritual Perspective Scale (SPS; Reed, 1987): a 10-item structured interview or questionnaire format administered to healthy and terminally ill adults. The measure has been shown to be reliable, accurate, and relevant in those populations.
- FACT-Sp (Fitchett, 2002): a 12-item scale that can be used alone or with the FACT-G, a general measure developed for cancer patients. Items examine faith and sense of purpose and meaning in life.

## References

Aday, R. (1984). Belief in afterlife and death anxiety: Correlates and comparisons. *Omega, 18*, 67–75.

Allport, G. W., & Ross, M. J. (1967). Personal religious orientation and prejudice. *Journal of Personality and Social Psychology, 5*, 432–443.

Batson, C. D., & Schoenrade, P. A. (1991a). Measuring religion as quest: 1) Validity concerns. *Journal for the Scientific Study of Religion, 30*, 416–429.

Batson, C. D., & Schoenrade, P. A. (1991b). Measuring religion as quest: 2) Reliability concerns. *Journal for the Scientific Study of Religion, 30*, 430–447.

Byock, I. R. (1995). *Missoula-VITAS quality of life index (version 25S)*. Miami, FL: VITAS Healthcare.

Chambers, L. W., Macdonald, L. A., Tugwell, P., Buchanan, W. W., & Kraag, G. (1982). The McMaster Health Index Questionnaire. *Journal of Rheumatology, 9*, 780–784.

Cohen, S. R., Mount, B. M., Strobel, M. G., & Bui, F. (1995). The McGill Quality of Life Questionnaire. *Palliative Medicine, 9*, 207–219.

Crumbaugh, J. (1977). The Seeking of Noetic Goals Test (SONG): A complementary scale to the Purpose in Life Test (PIL). *Journal of Clinical Psychology, 33*, 900–907.

Crumbaugh, J. C., & Maholick, L. T. (1964). An experimental study in existentialism: The psychometric approach to Frankl's concept of noogenic neurosis. *Journal of Clinical Psychology, 20,* 200–207.

Ferrans, C. E., & Powers, M. (1985). Quality of Life Index: Development and psychometric properties. *Advances in Nursing Science, 8*(1), 15–24.

Fitchett, G. (2002). *Assessing spiritual needs: A guide for caregivers.* Lima: Academic Renewal Press.

Gesser, G., Wong, P. T. P., & Reker, G. T. (1987). Death attitudes across the life span: Development and validation of the Death Attitude Profile. *Omega, 18*(2), 113–128.

Hood, R., & Morris, R. (1983). Toward a theory of death transcendence. *Journal for the Scientific Study of Religion, 22,* 353–365.

Kass, J., Friedman, R., Leserman, J., Zuttermeister, P., & Benson, H. (1991). Health outcomes and a new measure of spiritual experience. *Journal for the Scientific Study of Religion, 30,* 203–211.

Koenig, H., Cohen, H. J., Blazer, D. G., Pieper, C., Meador, K. G., Shelp, F., Goli, V., & DiPasquale, B. (1992). Religious coping and depression among elderly, hospitalized medically ill men. *American Journal of Psychiatry, 149,* 1693–1700.

MacAdam, D. B., & Smith, M. (1987). An initial assessment of suffering in terminal illness. *Palliative Medicine, 1,* 37–47.

McCanse, R. (1995). The McCanse Readiness for Death Instrument: A reliable and valid measure for hospice care. *Hospice Journal, 10*(1), 15–26.

McMillan, S. C., & Mahon, M. (1994). Measuring quality of life in hospice patients using a newly developed hospice quality of life index. *Quality of Life Research, 3,* 437–447.

Morris, J. N., Suissa, S., Sherwood, S., Wright, S. M., & Greer, D. (1986). Last days: A study of the quality of life of terminally ill cancer patients. *Journal of Chronic Diseases, 39*(1), 47–62.

Paloutzian, R. F., & Ellison, C. W. (1982). Loneliness, spiritual well-being and quality of life. In A. Peplau & D. Perlman (Eds.), *Loneliness: A sourcebook for current therapy* (pp. 224–237). Malden, MA: Wiley-Interscience.

Pargament, K. I., Ensing, D. S., Falgout, K., Olsen, H., Reilly, B., Van Haitsma, K., & Warren, R. (1990). God help me: (I): Religious coping efforts as predictors of the outcomes to significant negative life events. *American Journal of Community Psychology, 18,* 793–824.

Reed, P. (1987). Spirituality and well-being in terminally ill hospitalized adults. *Research in Nursing and Health, 10,* 335–344.

Reker, G., & Peacock, E. J. (1981). The Life Attitude Profile (LAP): A multidimensional instrument for assessing attitudes toward life. *Canadian Journal of Behavioural Science, 13,* 264–273.

Strayhorn, J. M., Weidman, C. S., & Larson, D. (1990). A measure of religiousness, and its relation to parent and child mental health variables. *Journal of Community Psychology, 18,* 34–43.

VandeCreek, L., Nye, C., & Herth, K. (1994). Where there's life, there's hope, and where there is hope, there is … *Journal of Religion and Health, 33*(1), 51–59.

Warner, S. C., & Williams, J. I. (1987). The Meaning in Life Scale: Determining the reliability and validity of a measure. *Journal of Chronic Diseases, 40,* 503–512.

# Appendix E
## Spiritual assessment resources

### Spiritual assessment: books and monographs

Fitchett, G. (1993, 2002). *Assessing spiritual needs: A guide for caregivers.* Lima, OH: Academic Renewal Press. (www.arpress.com, 1-800-537-1030)

Fitchett, G. (1993). *Spiritual assessment in pastoral care.* Decatur, GA: Journal of Pastoral Care Publications. This monograph, now out of print, describes and evaluates over 20 published models for spiritual assessment and history taking.

Hodge, D. R. (2003). *Spiritual assessment: Handbook for helping professionals.* Bolsford, CT: North American Association of Christians in Social Work. (www.nacsw.org)

Pruyser, P. W. (1976). *The minister as diagnostician.* Philadelphia: Westminster Press. This classic text sparked much of the work in this field. Pruyser's guidelines, or modified versions of them, are probably still the framework most frequently used by chaplains for spiritual assessment.

Ramsey, N. J. (1998). *Pastoral diagnosis: A resource for ministries of care and counseling.* Minneapolis, MN: Augsburg Fortress.

### Spiritual assessment: articles

Gaventa, W. C., Jr. (2001). Defining and assessing spirituality and spiritual supports: A rationale for inclusion in theory and practice. In W. C. Gaventa Jr. & D. L. Coulter (Eds.), *Spirituality and intellectual disability* (pp. 29–48). Binghamton, NY: Haworth Press.

Lewis, J. M. (2002). Pastoral assessment in hospital ministry: A conversational approach. *Chaplaincy Today, 18*(2), 5–3.

Lucas, A. M. (2001). Introduction to the discipline for pastoral care giving. In L. VandeCreek & A. M. Lucas (Eds.), *The discipline for pastoral care giving* (pp. 1–33). Binghamton, NY: Haworth Press.

Lyon, S. E. (2002). *Diaeresis and seven core needs: A model of spiritual assessment* (M. G. Montonye, Ed.). (Available from Martin G. Montonye, Hartford Hospital, 80 Seymour Street, Hartford, CT 06106.)

### Spiritual history taking: physician models

Anandarajah, G., & Hight, E. (2001). Spirituality and medical practice: Using the HOPE questions as a practical tool for spiritual assessment. *American Family Physician, 63*, 81–89.

Kuhn, C. C. (1988). A spiritual inventory of the medically ill patient. *Psychiatric Medicine, 6*(2), 87–100.

Maugans, T. A. (1996). The SPIRITual history. *Archives of Family Medicine, 5*, 11–16.

Puchalski, C., & Romer, A. L. (2000). Taking a spiritual history allows clinicians to understand patients more fully. *Journal of Palliative Medicine, 3*, 129–137. (Also see Puchalski's Website, www.gwish.org.)

## Nursing models

Carson, V. B. (Ed.). *Spiritual dimensions of nursing practice.* Philadelphia: W. B. Saunders.

Fish, S., & Shelly, J. A. (Eds.). (1978). *Spiritual care: The nurse's role.* Downers Grove, IL: Intervarsity Press.

# Appendix F
## Spirituality bibliography[1]

### *Christian Spirituality*, Volumes I, II, and III

These three works are volumes in the series *World Spirituality: An Encyclopedic History of the Religious Quest*. Chapters are arranged chronologically, with attention to movements, schools, orders, denominations, and geography, as appropriate. Noted scholars from each field author the appropriate chapters. Most essays assume the reader has at least a basic knowledge of church history. The three volumes on Christian spirituality include the following (chronologically):

McGinn, B., & Meyendorff, J. (Eds.). (1987). *Christian spirituality: Origins to the twelfth century*. New York: Crossroad. This is Volume 16 of *World Spirituality: An Encyclopedia History of the Religious Quest*.

Raitt, J. (Ed.). (1988). *Christian spirituality: High Middle Ages and Reformation*. New York: Crossroads. This is Volume 17 of *World Spirituality: An Encyclopedia History of the Religious Quest*.

Dupré, L., & Saliers, D. (Ed.). (1989). *Christian Spirituality: Post-Reformation and modern*. New York: Crossroad. This is Volume 18 of *World Spirituality: An Encyclopedia History of the Religious Quest*.

### Other works in the history of Christian spirituality

Calvin, J. (2001). *Writings on pastoral piety* (E. A. McKee, Ed.). New York: Paulist Press. This work presents the "other" side of Calvin—that is, the side generally not attended to until recent years. Here is Calvin's pastoral concern for the pious, ethical life grounded in prayer, worship, and the sacraments. Calvin's own words open up for the reader his sensitivity to the spiritual life as he asserts that prayer is the chief exercise of faith.

Edwards, J. (1994). *The religious affection*. Carlisle, PA: Banner of Truth Trust. Protestants with an interest in history and spiritual guidance will want to note Edwards's treatment of "distinguishing signs of truly gracious and holy affection." These signs are as valuable today as they were in 1746, when the work was first published.

Erb, P. C. (Ed.). (1983). *Pietists: Selected writings*. New York: Paulist Press. This book serves as a helpful introduction to selections of primary works from a number of pietists. Considerable attention is paid to Philip Jacob Spener, August Hermann Francke, and the Halle School. Those interested in Protestant spirituality will be well served by familiarity with these historical documents.

Hambrick-Stowe, C. E. (1982). *The practice of piety: Puritan devotional disciplines in seventeenth century New England.* Chapel Hill: University of North Carolina Press. The author opens up the world of Puritan spirituality in this work and in his book *Early New England Meditative Poetry: Anne Bradstreet and Edward Taylor.* Hambrick-Stowe reveals how the Reformed tradition as it was embodied by the Puritans' spirituality was a life-giving force seeking a better world.

Keller, R. S. (1992). *Georgia Harkness: For such a time as this.* Nashville, TN: Abingdon Press. This work is a biography of Georgia Harkness (1891–1974), who taught at Garrett Biblical Institute and the Pacific School of Religion. Described as the first woman to teach in a mainline Protestant seminary in the United States, Harkness raised prophetic and spiritual issues that remain crucial for a vision of the future.

Senn, F. (Ed.). (1986). *Protestant spiritual traditions.* New York: Paulist Press. Chapters introduce the spiritualities of the major Protestant traditions (e.g., Lutheran, Reformed, Anabaptist, Anglican, Puritan, Pietist, Methodist), with essays written by scholars in the field.

Sheldrake, P. (1995). *Spirituality and history: Questions of interpretation and method.* Maryknoll, NY: Orbis Books. Sheldrake, an Anglican scholar from Sarum College, Salisbury, England, is the current president of the Society for the Study for Christian Spirituality. In this work, he explores both the nature of history and the nature of spirituality. Two case studies serve to demonstrate his insights. He raises such questions as: Who creates or controls spirituality? Where are the groups that did not fit? How do historical models and typologies of spirituality shape our understanding?

Tyson, J. R. (Ed.). (1999). *An invitation to Christian spirituality: An ecumenical anthology.* New York: Oxford University Press. Tyson provides a historical introduction to spirituality by offering brief biographies of 76 key religious leaders and excerpts from their writings. Beginning with Ignatius of Antioch's *On Martyrdom* and Tertullilan of Carthage's *Jerusalem and Athens* and ending with Rosemary Radford Ruether's *Becoming a Feminist* and Desmond Tutu's *The Certainty of Freedom,* Tyson offers a comprehensive survey of the literature. Others included are Martin Luther, John Calvin, John and Charles Wesley, Jonathan Edwards, Horace Bushnell, Walter Rauschenbusch, Simone Weil, Howard Thurman, Martin Luther King Jr., James Cone, Mother Teresa, and Gustavo Gutierrez.

Wesley, J., & Wesley, C. (1981). *Selected prayers, hymns, journal notes, sermons, letters and treatises* (F. Whaling, Ed.). New York: Paulist Press. This book is a useful introduction to a variety of selections from the primary works of the Wesley brothers.

## Spirituality and health

Benson, H. (1996). *Timeless healing: The power and biology of belief.* New York: Fireside Books. Benson is an associate professor of medicine at Harvard Medical School and founder of Harvard's Mind/Body Medical Institute. He is also the author of *The Relaxation Response* and other works in the area of spirituality and health. Here, Benson essentially claims humans are "wired for God" and that this is good for us. This book provides a basic explication of his understanding of health and healing.

Borysenko, J. (1997). *Seven paths to God: The ways of the mystic.* Carlsbad, CA: Hay House. Borysenko was a founding director of the Mind/Body Institute, affiliated with Harvard University. This work is a very accessible description of seven different paths of faithfulness. Grounded in her own faith, Judaism, Borysenko's paths include elements from other religious traditions. This is perhaps most helpful in raising one's awareness of the variety of ways people can be faithful to God.

Dossey, L. (1997). *Be careful what you pray for … you just might get it.* San Francisco: Harper. In this work, Dossey explores the impact of negative intentions in nonlocal effects. He considers the question "Can prayer harm?" and includes contemporary scientific studies as evidence.

Dossey, L. (1999). *Reinventing medicine: Beyond mind-body to a new era of healing.* San Francisco: Harper. Dossey brings the insights of traditional Western medicine together with statistical studies involving intercessory prayer (nonlocal effects), prayer, dreams, and intuition for the purpose of reinventing medicine. He seeks to integrate ancient wisdom and modern medicine.

Downie, P. (1999). *Healing through prayer: Health practitioners tell the story.* Toronto: Anglican Book Centre. Twenty-six figures in the area of spirituality and health (including Larry Dossey, Herbert Benson, and Elisabeth Targ) reflect on their research and experience in the format of interviews. Chapters are divided into five major domains: science and spirituality, healing prayer in practice, the healing community, the perspective of other faiths, and a healing program at a local church. A 1-hour video featuring these interviews is also available from the Anglican Book Center, 600 Jarvis Street, Toronto, Ontario M4Y 2J6, Canada.

Flinders, C. L. (1999). *At the root of this longing: Reconciling a spiritual hunger and a feminist thirst.* San Francisco: Harper. Flinders draws on her knowledge of Julian of Norwich and other great female mystics to explore the tensions between the mystical path of silence, obedience, and the resistance of desires (often appropriate for men) and the spiritual needs of women for voice, selfhood, and reclaiming the body. Flinders is also the author of *Enduring Grace*, an exploration of the lives of female mystics.

Gottlieb, R. S. (1999). *A spirituality of resistance: Finding a peaceful heart and protecting the earth.* New York: Crossroad. Gottlieb attests that

> a spirituality of resistance, while recognizing the importance of working on ourselves, also directs us toward outer examination, outer transformation, and the pursuit of justice in the world … To find a peaceful heart, I will suggest, we need to live on this earth: fully conscious of what is happening on it, actively resisting that which we know to be evil or destructively ignorant.
>
> (p. 13)

He draws comparisons between the Holocaust and ecological destruction and warns that a psychic dependence on one's work can contribute to this ecocide.

## Spirituality and ministry

Bass, D. B. (2004). *The practicing congregation: Imagining a new Old Church.* Herndon, VA: Alban Institute. This work should be a key resource for mainline congregations who are interested in discovering the power of spiritual practices for congregational life. The notion of "retraditioning" addresses both the gifts of faith traditions and the life-giving energy of new ways of being together.

Bass, D. B. (2006). *Christianity for the rest of us: How the neighborhood church is transforming the faith.* San Francisco: HarperOne. This work explores mainline churches from a variety of denominations that are vital and lively communities. The book is a must-read for those who are searching for life-giving communities of faith.

Bass, D. C. (1998). *Practicing our faith: A way of life for a searching people.* San Francisco: Jossey Bass. This work broadens the understanding of spiritual practices to include such things as offering hospitality, singing, dying well, "saying 'yes,' saying 'no,'" giving testimony, and keeping the Sabbath. These practices are interpreted in ways that speak to people seeking to be faithful in the activity-filled, postmodern world.

Countryman, L. W. (1999). *Living on the border of the holy: Renewing the priesthood of all.* Harrisburg, PA: Morehouse. This book is an excellent resource for those seeking a renewed and creative understanding of priesthood (the gift given to all persons) or common ground for interfaith discussions.

Driskill, J. D. (1999). *Protestant spiritual exercises: Theology, history and practice.* Harrisburg, PA: Morehouse. The book includes a number of spiritual practices that have been used in Protestant traditions—for example, Martin Luther's four-stranded garland, the Puritans' interest in journals, and John and Charles Wesley's covenant groups. It includes a chapter on the responsible use of spiritual practices and an introduction to the spirituality that has characterized mainline Protestant churches. This book is also available in a Chinese edition from the Presbyterian Church of Taiwan.

Endo, S. (1980). *Silence.* New York: Taplinger. Endo's novel about a 17th-century Portuguese priest in Japan at a time of religious persecution raises many fundamental issues regarding the nature of Christ and the relationship between Christianity and culture.

Foster, R. J., & Yanni, K. A. (1992). *Celebrating the disciplines: A journal workbook to accompany celebration of discipline.* San Francisco: Harper. This workbook builds on Foster's earlier *Celebration of Discipline.* It provides an introduction to a number of spiritual practices associated with inward (e.g., prayer), outward (e.g., service), and corporate (e.g., worship) disciplines.

Hadaway, C. K., & Roozen, D. A. (1995). *Rerouting the Protestant mainstream: Sources of growth and opportunities for change.* Nashville, TN: Abingdon Press. Although it is a few years old, this work raises many significant questions that mainline churches must address if they are to thrive and be faithful to a renewal of their relationship with the holy.

Hamm, R. L. (2001). *2020 vision for the Christian church (Disciples of Christ).* St. Louis, MO: Chalice Press. Hamm provides a vision that includes a commitment to "true community, a deep Christian spirituality and a passion for justice." He demonstrates how the church of the future can embrace an experiential relationship with the divine both in the community of worship and in congregants' personal life.

Holmes, B. A. (2004). *Joy unspeakable: Contemplative practices of the Black church.* Minneapolis, MN: Augsburg Fortress. This work explores the notion of "contemplation" and demonstrates how the Black church embodies an understanding of contemplation that includes communal, active, verbal, and vocal dimensions of being with the holy. It helpfully challenges Eurocentric views that focus only on silence and quiet as contemplative practices.

Lebacqz, K., & Driskill, J. D. (2000). *Ethics and spiritual care: A guide for pastors, chaplains, and spiritual directors.* Nashville, TN: Abingdon Press. In this work, the authors explore the "muddy terrain" at the intersection of ethics and spiritual practice. They look at the contribution of a variety of ethical models for such practices as spiritual direction, pastoral care, spiritual guidance, and pastoral counseling. They also reflect on notions of "spiritual abuse" and "good spiritual care," noting the importance of the ministerial context for doing ministry.

Lee, U., Kim, J. H., Cho, M. J., Bass, D., & Pak, S. Y. (2005). *Singing the Lord's song in a new land: Korean American practices of faith.* Louisville, KY: Westminster/John Knox Press. A variety of Korean American spiritual practices are explored in this book. This work is a gift to all who seek to deepen their intercultural understanding of spiritual practices.

Matsuoka, F. (1998). *The color of faith: Building community in a multiracial society.* Cleveland, OH: United Church Press. When the not guilty verdict was rendered in the O. J. Simpson trial, racial divisions within the United States stood in stark relief. Why did diverse racial communities understand this trial from such differing perspectives? Matsuoka explores this question and looks at its implications for the future of religious communities in the United States.

Miller, W. R. (Ed.). (1999). *Integrating spirituality into treatment: Resource for practitioners.* Washington, DC: American Psychological Association. Chapters address such issues as spirituality and health, assessment, meditation, prayer, and values. Spiritual issues in treatment include surrender, acceptance and forgiveness, and hope. This is a useful resource on spirituality for counselors from various disciplines.

Sadler, K. M. (Ed.). (2001). *The book of daily prayer: Morning and evening.* Cleveland, OH: Pilgrim Press. Scripture readings and prayers for morning and evening are provided for each day of 2002 by a variety of pastors, administrators, and academics primarily (but not exclusively) from the United Church of Christ.

Thompson, M. J. (1995). *Soul feast: An invitation to the Christian spiritual life.* Louisville, KY: Westminster/John Knox Press. This is a highly used resource for fostering spiritual development in congregational life. Thompson explores such topics as worship, fasting, prayer, hospitality, and spiritual direction and provides suggestions for their significance and use in the church.

Thurman, H. (1979). *With head and heart.* San Diego, CA: Harcourt Brace Jovanovich. This is a stunning autobiography of one of America's great religious leaders. Thurman's reflections on his experiences as an African American leader expose not only the depth of his spirituality but also the forces of racism and oppression with which he had to contend.

Washington, J. M. (1994). *Conversations with God: Two centuries of prayers by African Americans.* San Francisco: Harper Collins. This is an anthology of prayers from a "determined yet degraded people," as Cornel West put it. Through these prayers, one enters the rich depth of African American spirituality.

Wicks, R. J. (Ed.). (1995). *Handbook of spirituality for ministers.* New York: Paulist Press. This work serves as a helpful resource for clergy who wish to integrate increased spiritual depth into their ministerial practices. Thirty-five short essays address such issues as spiritual guidance, prayer, social justice, psychology, the spirituality of the minister, ministering to persons with HIV/AIDS, spirituality in ministry to Hispanics, and African American spirituality.

Wicks, R. J. (Ed.). (2000). *Handbook of spirituality for ministers* (Vol. 2). New York: Paulist Press. This edited work includes chapters largely—although not exclusively—written by Roman Catholic theologians, including William A. Barry, Janet Ruffing, Keith J. Egan, Margaret Guenther, E. Glenn Hinson, Kathleen Fischer, and Thomas Hart. Topics include scripture, prayer, justice, darkness and hope, spiritual direction, and mentoring.

144 *Appendix F*

## Spiritual direction and pastoral care

Bidwell, D. R. (2004). *Short-term spiritual guidance.* Minneapolis, MN: Augsburg Fortress. Working from a Protestant context, the author explores the importance of short-term pastoral encounters as opportunities for providing spiritual guidance. Bidwell knows the research on short-term pastoral counseling and explores the additional possibilities that such encounters provide for spiritual care.

Ferris, M. (1993). *Compassioning: Basic counselling skills for Christian care-givers.* Kansas City, MO: Sheed and Ward. By integrating theological and psychological insights, Ferris extends the active listening and counseling scales of George Gazda to teach spiritually informed pastoral counseling. Practical exercises are provided for improving one's active listening skills.

Fitchett, G. (1993). *Assessing spiritual needs: A guide for caregivers.* Minneapolis, MN: Augsburg Fortress. Fitchett discusses the importance of spiritual assessment in pastoral ministry and provides a description of the $7 \times 7$ model for spiritual assessment. After providing a set of guidelines for evaluating the strengths and weaknesses of various models of spiritual assessment, he evaluates the spiritual assessment models of Paul Pruyser and Elisabeth McSherry and the diagnostic category of "spiritual distress" of the North American Nursing Diagnosis Association.

Ramsey, N. J. (1998). *Pastoral diagnosis: A resource for ministries of care and counseling.* Minneapolis, MN: Augsburg Fortress. Ramsey defines diagnosis as a hermeneutical process "reflecting the values and assumptions of the perspectives of the practitioner" (p. 4). Tackling issues of pastoral identity and pastoral diagnosis and placing them in the context of theological and ethical reflection opens up opportunities for redemptive transformation that can be provided by informed pastoral practice.

Richards, P. S., & Bergin, A. E. (1997). *A spiritual strategy for counseling and psychotherapy.* Washington, DC: American Psychological Association. This well-researched work seeks to integrate a theistic spiritual strategy into mainstream approaches to psychotherapy. It will be of interest to pastoral counselors and clinically trained therapists who want to integrate spirituality into their counseling. The authors—with doctorates from the University of Minnesota and Stanford University, respectively—teach in the psychology department at Brigham Young University.

Ruffing, J. (2000). *Spiritual direction: Beyond the beginnings.* New York: Paulist Press. Although a number of works provide an introduction to spiritual direction, Ruffing has given us a volume that assumes the basics and accordingly illuminates themes and offers insights that are especially helpful to the experienced spiritual director.

Smith, A., Jr. (1997). *Navigating the deep river: Spirituality in African American families.* Cleveland, OH: United Church Press. Smith presents a context-sensitive systems approach to African American families that discloses the way the spiritual life of the African American community is infused throughout pastoral practices and activities. Discovering and navigating the deep river yields helpful insights for all who are concerned about the quality of caring on and for the planet.

Stairs, J. (2000). *Listening for the soul: Pastoral care and spiritual direction.* Minneapolis, MN: Augsburg Fortress. This work is a careful exploration of the pastoral opportunities afforded by pastoral care, pastoral counseling, and spiritual direction. Stairs is careful to delineate the common ground and the distinctive attributes of each mode of ministry. People who provide spiritual direction and pastoral counseling need to be aware of the ethical boundaries and praxis aspects Stairs identifies.

Vest, N. (Ed.). (2000). *Still listening: New horizons in spiritual direction.* Harrisburg, PA: Morehouse. This book features essays of interest to spiritual directors who are working with traumatized persons, church dropouts, people living with economic poverty, and the dying as well as to those providing guidance in the business world. Contributors include Margaret Guenther, Kenneth Leech, Janet Ruffing, Joseph Driskill, Norvene Vest, and Howard Rice.

## Note

1 Reprinted with permission, Joseph Driskill, Associate Professor of Spirituality, Pacific School of Religion, 1798 Avenue, Berkeley, CA 94709, 2004.

# Appendix G
## BMMRS

**Brief Multidimensional Measure of Religiousness/
Spirituality**[1]

To assess the relationship between spirituality and religiousness, the Fetzer Institute and the National Institute on Aging Working Group (1999) developed a set of measurement items divided into domains. The result was the Brief Multidimensional Measure of Religiousness/Spirituality (BMMRS), a tool for researchers measuring spirituality and religiousness from a multidimensional approach. The measure was embedded in the 1997–1998 General Social Survey (GSS), a random national survey of the National Data Program for the Social Sciences. The basic purpose of the GSS was to gather and disseminate data on contemporary American society to monitor and explain trends in attitudes and behaviors and to compare the United States to other societies. The assessment and the results of the survey are in a booklet that can be obtained from the Fetzer Institute's website (www.fetzer.org). A booklet describes the BMMRS (which also can be obtained on the Fetzer Institute's website) and contains the Daily Spiritual Experience Scale (DSES; Underwood & Teresi, 2002), along with information about development, reliability, exploratory factor analyses, and preliminary construct validity of the BMMRS. Researchers interested in the statistical data should consult the booklet. According to the Fetzer Institute (1999), "the results to date support the theoretical basis of the measure and indicate it has the … reliability and validity to facilitate further research" (p. 89). The items from the DSES were also included in the 2002 GSS.

The Fetzer Institute and the National Institute on Aging Working Group identified 12 domains as essential for studies in which some measure of health serves as an outcome, and they structured the BMMRS on the basis of these domains. They chose these domains because of the strength of their conceptualization and their theoretical or empirical connection to health outcomes. The domains are as follows:

- Daily Spiritual Experiences
- Meaning
- Values

- Beliefs
- Forgiveness
- Private Religious Practices
- Religious/Spiritual Coping
- Religious Support
- Religious/Spiritual History
- Commitment
- Organizational Religiousness
- Religious Preference.

The assessment has a short form and a long form. Because some domains are not included in the short form, the long form is presented here. The material is taken directly from the BMMRS unless otherwise indicated.

The first domain is intended to measure the person's perception of the transcendent being (God, the divine) in daily life and perception of interaction with or involvement of the transcendent in life. The items attempt to measure experience rather than cognitive constructions. This domain makes spirituality its central focus and can be used effectively across many religious boundaries (Fetzer Institute, 1999, p. 11).

## Daily spiritual experiences

### *Connection with the transcendent (Fetzer Institute, 1999, p. 12)*

1  I feel God's presence.
2  I experience a connection to all of life.

As in people's relationships with each other, this quality of intimacy with God can be important. These questions were developed to address both people whose experience of relationship with the transcendent being is one of personal intimacy and those who describe a more general sense of unity as their connection with the transcendent being.

### *Transcendent sense of self (Fetzer Institute, 1999, p. 13)*

3  During worship, or at other times when connecting with God, I feel intense joy which lifts me out of my daily concerns.

This item attempts to identify the experience of a lively worship service during which one's day-to-day concerns can dissolve. People may also be able to transcend the difficulties of present physical ills or psychological situations through an awareness that life consists of more than the physical and psychological realm.

### Sense of support from the transcendent (Fetzer Institute, 1999, p. 12)

A sense of support is expressed in three ways: strength and comfort, perceived love, and inspiration/discernment.

  4  I find strength in my religion or spirituality.
  5  I find comfort in my religion or spirituality.

This dimension has been described as "social support from God." The items are intended to measure a direct sense of support and comfort from the transcendent (p. 13).

### Sense of wholeness, internal integration (Fetzer Institute, 1999, p. 13)

  6  I feel deep inner peace or harmony.

This item attempts to move beyond mere psychological well-being. It implies the sense of wholeness people may feel while experiencing adverse circumstances. Respondents may believe that integration of experiences is possible despite the challenges they face. The word *deep* allows people to consider factors other than psychological ease such as interpeace.

### Inspiration/discernment (Fetzer Institute, 1999, p. 13)

  7  I ask for God's help in the midst of daily activities.
  8  I feel guided by God in the midst of daily activities.

These items address the expectation of divine intervention or inspiration and a sense that a divine force has intervened or inspired. The *guidance* item was most often deemed similar to a "nudge" from God and more rarely as a more dramatic action.

### Perceived love (Fetzer Institute, 1999, p. 13)

  9  I feel God's love for me directly.
 10  I feel God's love for me through others.

Individuals can believe that God is loving without feeling loved themselves. The emotional support of feeling loved may prove important in the relationship of religious spiritual issues to health outcomes. The quality of love imputed to God has potential differences from the love humans give each other, and there is a kind of love from others that many people attribute to God. God's love can be experienced as affirming and can contribute to self-confidence and a sense of self-worth independent of actions.

## *Sense of awe (Fetzer Institute, 1999, p. 13)*

11    I am spiritually touched by the beauty of creation.

This dimension attempts to capture the ways in which people experience the transcendent. A sense of awe can be provoked be exposure to nature, human beings, or the night sky and elicit experiences of the spiritual that crosses religious boundaries and affect people who have no religious connection.

## *Sense of gratitude (Fetzer Institute, 1999, p. 13)*

12    I feel thankful for my blessings.

This aspect of spirituality is considered central by many people and has potential to psychologically positive ways of viewing life. Because of the potential connections between gratitude and circumstances of life, external stressors may modify a respondent's feelings of thankfulness. It is important to note, however, that some people find blessings even in the most dire circumstances.

## *Sense of compassion (Fetzer Institute, 1999, p. 14)*

13    I feel a selfless caring for others.

People of different cultures understand selfless caring. Compassion is valued in Buddhist, Christian, Jewish, and other traditions and may be a useful measure.

## *Sense of mercy (Fetzer Institute, 1999, p. 14)*

14    I accept others even when they do things I think are wrong.

This item addresses the felt sense of mercy, rather than the mere cognitive awareness that mercy is a good quality. This measure was successful in presenting mercy as a neutral, easily understood concept. Mercy is ... closely linked to forgiveness but is a deeper experience than isolated acts of forgiveness.

## *Longing for the transcendent (Fetzer Institute, 1999, p. 14)*

15    I desire to be closer to God or in union with Him.
16    In general, how close to God do you feel?

People administering the questionnaire should always pair teams 15 and 16 to fully evaluate the concept of longing. There are two opposite ways of responding to Item 15: some people feel they are so close to God that it is not possible to get closer; others have no desire to become closer. Question16 assesses the respondent's current degree of intimacy or connection with God.

## Meaning (Fetzer Institute, 1999, p. 21)

"Constructing meaning from life events is an essentially human endeavor. Less clear is the means of measuring a person's search for meaning (the process) and the success or failure of that search (the outcome)." Attempts to measure the construct of meaning grow largely out of the theoretical work of Viktor Frankl (1946/1959), who asserted that the "will to meaning" (p. 154) is an essential human characteristic, and physical and mental symptomatology can result when it is blocked or unfulfilled" (p. 19). The search for meaning has also been defined as one of the critical functions of religion. Frankl (1946/1959) himself viewed meaning in religious terms. Meaning as he saw it was something to "discover rather than or invent" (p. 113) that is, every individual has a unique, externally given purpose in life (p 19).

### *Meaning—long form (Fetzer Institute, 1999, p. 21)*

Instructions: Please circle how much you agree or disagree with the following statements on the scale below.

1—Strongly disagree; 2—Disagree; 3—Neutral; 4—Agree; 5—Strongly agree

1   My spiritual beliefs give meaning to my life's joys and sorrows.
2   The goals of my life grow out of my understanding of God.
3   Without a sense of spirituality, my daily life would be meaningless.
4   The meaning in my life comes from feeling connected to other living things.
5   My religious beliefs help me find a purpose in even the most painful and confusing events in my life.
6   When I lose touch with God, I have a harder time feeling that there is purpose and meaning in life.
7   My spiritual beliefs give my life a sense of significance and purpose.
8   My mission in life is guided/shaped by my faith in God.
9   When I am disconnected from the spiritual dimension of my life, I lose my sense of purpose.
10   My relationship with God helps me find meaning in the ups and downs of life.
11   My life is significant because I am part of God's plan.
12   What I try to do in my day-to-day life is important to me from a spiritual point of view.
13   I am trying to fulfill my God-given purpose in life.
14   Knowing that I am a part of something greater than myself gives meaning to my life.
15   Looking at the most troubling or confusing events from a spiritual perspective adds meaning to my life.
16   My purpose in life reflects what I believe God wants for me.
17   Without my religious foundation, my life would be meaningless.

18 My feelings of spirituality add meaning to the events in my life.
19 God plays a role in how I choose my path in life.
20 My spirituality helps define the goals I set for myself.

## Values (Fetzer Institute, 1999, p. 25)

This domain is intended to measure dimensions distinct from the value the individual places on religion. This domain is not about the sheer presence or absence of values per se; everyone values something. Instead, it is based on values as goals and on norms as the means to those goals. This domain attempts to assess the extent to which a person's behavior reflects a normative expression of faith or religion as the ultimate value.

### *Values—short form*

Instructions: Please circle how much you agree or disagree with the following statements on the scale below.

1—Strongly disagree; 2—Disagree; 3—Neutral; 4—Agree; 5—Strongly agree

1 My whole approach to life is based on my religion.
2 Although I believe in my religion, many other things are more important in life.
3 My faith helps me know right from wrong.

## Beliefs (Fetzer Institute, 1999, p. 31)

The central feature of religiousness is the cognitive dimension of belief; members of religious groups are identified as "believers." However, members of the same religious group vary in the strength of their belief and may also disagree about what their beliefs should be. By definition, beliefs differ from religion to religion, so finding beliefs that religions might have in common with spirituality is, by definition, impossible.

Beliefs can be central to health and healing as well. The placebo effect, a change in a patient's condition attributable to the symbolic import of a treatment rather than to a specific pharmacological or physiological intervention, has long been acknowledged. Benson (1996) argued that religious faith mobilizes placebo effects by enhancing the memory of repeated, familiar, positive therapeutic states. Beliefs about the meaning of suffering and death are in some way central to all religions; they create webs of meaning and comprehensibility that may comfort and sustain believers, even in the midst of acute tragedy or long-term suffering.

### Beliefs—long form (short form not included)

1   How much is religion a source of strength and comfort to you? (Yale Health and Aging Project)

    1   None        2   A little        3   A great deal

2   Do you believe there is a life after death? (GSS, 1968)

    1   Yes        2   No        3   Undecided

Instructions: Please circle how much you agree or disagree with the following statements on the scale below.

1—Strongly disagree; 2—Disagree; 3—Neutral; 4—Agree; 5—Strongly agree

3   God's goodness and love are greater than we can possibly imagine.
4   Despite all the things that go wrong, the world is still moved by love.
5   When faced with a tragic event I try to remember that God still loves me and that there is hope for the future.
6   I feel that it is important for my children to believe in God.
7   I think that everything that happens has a purpose.

## Forgiveness (Fetzer Institute, 1999, pp. 35–36)

This domain includes five dimensions of forgiveness: making confession, feeling forgiven by God, feeling forgiven by others, forgiving others, and forgiving oneself. The concept of forgiveness is central to the Judeo-Christian tradition. It is the focus of a major Jewish holiday (Yom Kippur) and is a theme in much of Jewish scripture. It is also the core belief of the Christian faith; it is celebrated at Easter, the most important Christian holiday. Jews and Christians have concepts of both divine and interpersonal forgiveness, the latter modeled on the former. The items below can be self-administered or administered by phone or in person. These items assess current behavior and attitudes and cannot predict future behavior.

### Forgiveness—long form

*Confession*

1   It is easy for me to admit that I am wrong (Mauger, Freeman, Grove, McBridge, & McKinney, 1992)

    1   Always or almost always
    2   Often
    3   Seldom
    4   Never

2   If I hear a sermon, I usually think about things that I have done wrong (Mauger et al., 1992).

　　1   Always or almost always
　　2   Often
　　3   Seldom
　　4   Never

## Forgiveness by God

3   I believe that God has forgiven me for things I have done wrong.

　　1   Always or almost always
　　2   Often
　　3   Seldom
　　4   Never

4   I believe that there are times when God has punished me.

　　1   Always or almost always
　　2   Often
　　3   Seldom
　　4   Never

## Forgiveness by others

5   I believe that when people say they forgive me for something I did they really mean it (Mauger et al., 1992).

　　1   Always or almost always
　　2   Often
　　3   Seldom
　　4   Never

6   I often feel that no matter what I do now I will never make up for the mistakes I have made in the past (Mauger et al., 1992).

　　1   Always or almost always
　　2   Often
　　3   Seldom
　　4   Never

## Forgiveness of others

7   I am able to make up pretty easily with friends who have hurt me in some way (Mauger et al., 1992).

　　1   Always or almost always
　　2   Often

3   Seldom

4   Never

8   I have grudges, which I have held onto for months or years (Mauger et al., 1992).

1   Always or almost always

2   Often

3   Seldom

4   Never

## Forgiveness of oneself

9   I find it hard to forgive myself for some things that I have done (Mauger et al., 1992).

1   Always or almost always

2   Often

3   Seldom

4   Never

10   I often feel like I have failed to live the right kind of life (Mauger et al., 1992).

1   Always or almost always

2   Often

3   Seldom

4   Never

## Forgiveness—short form

1   I have forgiven myself for things that I have done wrong.

1   Always or almost always

2   Often

3   Seldom

4   Never

2   I have forgiven those who hurt me.

1   Always or almost always

2   Often

3   Seldom

4   Never

3   I know that God forgives me.

1   Always or almost always

2   Often

3   Seldom

4   Never

## Private religious practice (Fetzer Institute, 1999, p. 39)

These items are designed to assess private religious and spiritual practices, a conceptual domain or dimension of religious involvement often characterized by terms such as *non-organizational, informal,* and *non-institutional religiosity.* Private religious practices represent a subset of behaviors constituting the larger construct of religious involvement. The domain of private religious practices is distinct from the domain of public (i.e., organizational, formal, institutional) religious behavior. Private practices are non-organizational in that they take place outside the context of organized religion. They are informal in that they may not always occur at fixed times or in fixed places or necessarily involve fixed liturgical formulas. Finally, they are non-institutional in that they are private behaviors that occur at home—individually or in a family setting—rather than as collective experiences in a formal place of worship.

### *Private religious practices—long form*

1  How often do you pray privately in places other than at church or synagogue?

|   |   |   |   |
|---|---|---|---|
| 1 | Several times a day | 5 | A few times a month |
| 2 | Once a day | 6 | Once a month |
| 3 | A few times a week | 7 | Less than once a month |
| 4 | Once a week | 8 | Never |

2  How often do you watch or listen to religious programs on TV or radio?

|   |   |   |   |
|---|---|---|---|
| 1 | Several times a day | 5 | A few times a month |
| 2 | Once a day | 6 | Once a month |
| 3 | A few times a week | 7 | Less than once a month |
| 4 | Once a week | 8 | Never |

3  How often do you read the Bible or other religious literature?

|   |   |   |   |
|---|---|---|---|
| 1 | Several times a day | 5 | A few times a month |
| 2 | Once a day | 6 | Once a month |
| 3 | A few times a week | 7 | Less than once a month |
| 4 | Once a week | 8 | Never |

4  How often are prayers or grace said before or after meals in your home?

|   |   |   |   |
|---|---|---|---|
| 1 | At all meals | 3 | At least once a week |
| 2 | Once a day | 4 | Never |

## Religious/spiritual coping (Fetzer Institute, 1999, pp. 43–45)

The items in this domain of the BMMRS assess two patterns of religious/spiritual coping with stressful life events: positive religious and spiritual coping, reflective of benevolent religious methods of understanding and dealing with life stressors, and negative religious/spiritual coping, reflective of religious struggle. Empirical studies have shown a clear connection between stressful life events and various forms of religious/spiritual involvement (Bearon & Koenig, 1990; Bjorck & Cohen, 1993; Ellison & Taylor 1996; Lindenthal, Myers, Pepper, & Stein, 1970). Major life events can threaten or harm objects of significance—the sense of meaning, intimacy with others, personal control, physical health, or sense of personal comfort, etc. Religion (defined broadly as the search for significance in ways related to the sacred) offers a variety of coping methods for conserving these objects of significance in times of stress or, if that is no longer possible, transforming these objects of significance (Pargament, 1997).

The BMMRS uses five approaches to measure religious and spiritual coping: the indicators approach, the overall approach, the general coping approach, the patterns of religious coping approach, and the specific religious coping methods approach.

- The *indicators approach* uses global religious items (e.g., frequency of prayer or frequency of church attendance) as indicators of religious/spiritual coping. Evidence shows that measures of religious/spiritual coping methods predict outcomes more strongly than do religious indicators.
- The *overall approach* assesses overall degree of religious and spiritual involvement in coping. The BMMRS draws items from the Religious Coping Index (Koenig et al., 1993) for this approach.
- The *general coping approach* items reflect a few uses of religion in the process of coping with a life stressor. An example is the Way of Coping Scale (Lazarus & Fokman, 1984).
- The BMMRS items measure the *patterns of religious coping* approach in terms of what people generally do when they face stressors or what they do when they face a particular stressor. The subscale of the COPE Inventory taps into an emotion-focused, spiritually based coping method. The BMMRS draws four items from this subscale.
- The *specific religious coping methods* approach assumes that religion offers a variety of methods for coping with life's problems and that it should be possible to assess those methods in detail. Several approaches have been used to measure specific methods of religious/spiritual coping. Two such approaches are to assess styles of religious problem solving and assess religious coping activities (RCA). There are three religious styles of problem solving:

  1  Deferring style—control is sought from God and places the responsibility for coping on God.
  2  Collaborative style—control is sought with God and the individual and God shares the responsibility for coping.
  3  Self-directing style—control rests within the individual; the individual, takes the responsibility for coping himself/herself.

The items cover various domains of the problem-solving process: problem definition, generation of alternative solutions, selection of a solution, implementation of the solution, conclusion, and redefinition of the problem.

The RCA items measure a wide range of religious and spiritual coping methods. They were developed through a literature review and interviews with clergy and lay adults who were dealing with various crises. Studies have shown that scores on the RCA scales are predictors of mood, depression, anxiety, and religious outcomes among people facing various crises (Pargament, 1997). These predictors are consistent with symptoms of a spiritual crisis.

The Revised COPE Inventory (RCOPE) (Pargament & Koenig, 1997) is designed to examine the positive and negative sides of religious and spiritual coping. It includes five items and three item versions that assess 17 religious and spiritual coping methods. These coping methods are targeted to the search for meaning, intimacy, self-development, comfort, and spirituality.

### Religious/spiritual coping—long form

Asterisks indicate that the item is on the third item version of the given subscale.

### Brief RCOPE items (Pargament, Smith, Koenig, & Perez, 1989)

Instructions (Dispositional): Think about how you try to understand and deal with major problems in your life. To what extent is each involved in the way you cope?

#### Positive religious/spiritual coping subscale

1  I think about how my life is part of a larger spiritual force (search for spiritual connection).* [*item is on the three-item version of the given subscale]

|   |             |   |            |
|---|-------------|---|------------|
| 1 | A great deal | 2 | Quite a bit |
| 3 | Somewhat     | 4 | Not at all  |

2  I work together with God as a partner to get through hard times (collaborative religious coping).*

|   |             |   |            |
|---|-------------|---|------------|
| 1 | A great deal | 2 | Quite a bit |
| 3 | Somewhat     | 4 | Not at all  |

3  I look to God for strength, support, and guidance in crises (seeking spiritual support).*

|   |             |   |            |
|---|-------------|---|------------|
| 1 | A great deal | 2 | Quite a bit |
| 3 | Somewhat     | 4 | Not at all  |

4  I try to find the lesson from God in crises (benevolent religious appraisal).

|   |             |   |            |
|---|-------------|---|------------|
| 1 | A great deal | 2 | Quite a bit |
| 3 | Somewhat     | 4 | Not at all  |

5    I confess my sins and ask for God's forgiveness (ritual purification).

    1    A great deal               2    Quite a bit
    3    Somewhat                4    Not at all

*Negative religious/spiritual coping subscale*

1    I feel that stressful situations are God's way of punishing me for my sins or lack of spirituality (punishing God reappraisal).*

    1    A great deal               2    Quite a bit
    3    Somewhat                4    Not at all

2    I wonder whether God has abandoned me (spiritual discontent).*

    1    A great deal               2    Quite a bit
    3    Somewhat                4    Not at all

3    I try to make sense of the situation and decide what to do without relying on God (self-directed religious coping).*

    1    A great deal               2    Quite a bit
    3    Somewhat                4    Not at all

4    I question whether God really exists (religious doubts).

    1    A great deal               2    Quite a bit
    3    Somewhat                4    Not at all

5    I express anger at God for letting terrible things happen (anger at God).

    1    A great deal               2    Quite a bit
    3    Somewhat                4    Not at all

*Overall religious and spiritual coping item*

To what extent is your religion involved in understanding or dealing with stressful situations in any way?*

    1    Very involved             2    Somewhat involved
    3    Not very involved        4    Not involved at all

## Note

1 Reprinted from *Multidimensional Measurement of Religious/Spirituality for Use in Health Research* (pp. 1–96), by the Fetzer Institute and the National Institute on Aging Working Group, 2007, available at www.fetzer.org. Copyright 2007 Lynn G. Underwood, professor of biomedical humanities and director, Center for Literature, Medicine and Biomedical Humanities, Hiram College.

# References

Bearon, L., & Koenig, G. (1990). Religious cognition and use of prayer in health and illness. *Gerontologist, 30*, 249–253.

Benson, H. (1996). Timeless healing: The power and biology of belief. New York: Simon & Schuster.

Bjorck, J., & Cohen, H. (1993). Coping with threats, losses and challenges. *Journal of Social and Clinical Psychology, 12*, 36–72.

Ellison, C., & Taylor, J. (1996). Turning to prayer: Social and situational antecedents of religious coping among African Americans. *Review of Religious Research, 38*, 61–81.

Fetzer Institute/National Institute on Aging Working Group. (1999). Multidimensional measurement of religiousness/spirituality for use in health research: A report of the Fetzer Institute/National Institute on Aging Working Group. Kalamazoo, MI.

Frankl, V. E. (1946/1959). *Man's search for meaning: An introduction to logotherapy.* Boston: Beacon Press.

General Social Survey (GSS). (1990) Principal investigators J. Davis, T. Smith, & P. Marsdan. Funded by the National Science Foundation, National Opinion Research Center, Ann Arbor, MI.

Koenig, H., Cohen, J. J., Blazer, D. G., Pieper, C., Meador, K. G., Shelp, F., Goli, V., & DiPasquale, B. (1993). Religious coping and depression among elderly hospitalized medically ill men. *American Journal of Psychiatry, 149*, 1693–1700.

Lazarus, R., & Folkman, S. (1984). *Stress, appraisal and coping.* New York: Springer.

Lindenthal, J., Myers, J., Pepper, M., & Stein, M (1970). Mental status and religious behaviour. *Journal for the Scientific Study of Religion, 9*, 143–149.

Mauger, P., Freeman, P., Grove, D., McBridge A., & McKinney K. (1992). The measurement of forgiveness: Preliminary research. *Journal of Psychology and Christianity, 11*(2), 170–180.

Pargament, K. (1997). *The psychology of religion and coping: Theory, research, practice.* New York: Guilford Press.

Pargament, K., & Koenig, H. (1997). A comprehensive measure of religious coping: Development and initial validation of the RCOPE. Report presented at the Retirement Research Foundation, Chicago, IL.

Pargament, K., Smith, B., Koenig, H., & Perez, L. (1989). Patterns of positive and negative religious coping with major life stressors. *Journal for the Scientific Study of Religion, 37*(4), 711–725.

Underwood, L. G., & Teresi, J. A. (2002) The daily spiritual experience scale: Development, theoretical description, reliability, exploratory factor analysis, and preliminary construct validity using health-related data. *Annals of Behavioral Medicine, 24*(1), 22–33.

# Appendix H

## Revised Coping Method (RCOPE)

The Revised COPE Inventory (RCOPE) (Pargament & Koenig, 1997) is designed to examine the positive and negative sides of religious and spiritual coping. It includes five items and three item versions that assess 17 religious and spiritual coping methods. These coping methods are targeted to the search for meaning, intimacy, self-development, comfort, and spirituality.

### Religious/spiritual coping—long form

Asterisks indicate that the item is on the third item version of the given subscale.

*Brief RCOPE items (Pargament, Smith, Koenig, & Perez, 1998)*

Instructions (Dispositional): Think about how you try to understand and deal with major problems in your life. To what extent is each involved in the way you cope?

*Positive religious/spiritual coping subscale*

1  I think about how my life is part of a larger spiritual force (search for spiritual connection).* [*item is on the three-item version of the given subscale]

   | 1 | A great deal | 2 | Quite a bit |
   |---|---|---|---|
   | 3 | Somewhat | 4 | Not at all |

2  I work together with God as a partner to get through hard times (collaborative religious coping).*

   | 1 | A great deal | 2 | Quite a bit |
   |---|---|---|---|
   | 3 | Somewhat | 4 | Not at all |

3  I look to God for strength, support, and guidance in crises (seeking spiritual support).*

   | 1 | A great deal | 2 | Quite a bit |
   |---|---|---|---|
   | 3 | Somewhat | 4 | Not at all |

4    I try to find the lesson from God in crises (benevolent religious appraisal).

    1    A great deal              2    Quite a bit
    3    Somewhat                  4    Not at all

5    I confess my sins and ask for God's forgiveness (ritual purification).

    1    A great deal              2    Quite a bit
    3    Somewhat                  4    Not at all

## *Negative religious/spiritual coping subscale*

1    I feel that stressful situations are God's way of punishing me for my sins or lack of spirituality (punishing God reappraisal).*

    1    A great deal              2    Quite a bit
    3    Somewhat                  4    Not at all

2    I wonder whether God has abandoned me (spiritual discontent).*

    1    A great deal              2    Quite a bit
    3    Somewhat                  4    Not at all

3    I try to make sense of the situation and decide what to do without relying on God (self-directed religious coping).*

    1    A great deal              2    Quite a bit
    3    Somewhat                  4    Not at all

4    I question whether God really exists (religious doubts).

    1    A great deal              2    Quite a bit
    3    Somewhat                  4    Not at all

5    I express anger at God for letting terrible things happen (anger at God).

    1    A great deal              2    Quite a bit
    3    Somewhat                  4    Not at all

## *Overall religious and spiritual coping item*

To what extent is your religion involved in understanding or dealing with stressful situations in any way?*

    1    Very involved             2    Somewhat involved
    3    Not very involved         4    Not involved at all

## RCOPE subscales and items and definitions of religious and spiritual coping methods

### *Religious and spiritual methods of coping to find meaning*

Instructions: The following items deal with ways you coped with the negative event in your life. There are many ways to try to deal with problems. These items ask what you did to cope with this negative event. Obviously different people deal with things in different ways, but we are interested in how you tried to deal with it. Each item says something about a particular way of coping. We want to know to what extent you did what the item says. How much or how frequently? Don't answer on the basis of what worked or not, just whether or not you did it. Use these raceway choices. Try to rate each item separately in your mind from the others. Make your answers as true FOR YOU as you can. Circle the answer that best applies to you.

1—Not at all; 2—Somewhat; 3—Quite a bit; 4—A great deal

### *Benevolent Religious Reappraisal—redefining the stressor through religion as benevolent and potentially beneficial*

1    Saw my situation as part of God's plan.*
2    Tried to find a lesson from God in the event.*
3    Tried to see how God might be trying to strengthen me in this situation.*
4    Thought that the event might bring me closer to God.*

### *Punishing God Reappraisal—redefining the stressor as a punishment from God for the person's sins*

1    Wondered what I did for God to punish me.*
2    Decided that God was punishing me for my sins.*
3    Felt punished by God for my lack of devotion.*
4    Wondered if God allowed this event to happen to me because of my sins.*
5    Wondered whether God was punishing me because of my lack of faith.*

### *Demonic Reappraisal—redefining the stressor as an act of the Devil*

1    Believed the Devil was responsible for my situation.*
2    Felt the situation was the work of the Devil.*
3    Felt the Devil was trying to turn me away from God.*
4    Decided the Devil made this happen.*
5    Wondered if the Devil had anything to do with this situation.*

***Reappraisal of God's powers***—*redefining God's power to influence the stressful situation*

1   Questioned the power of God.*
2   Thought that some things are beyond God's control.*
3   Realized that God cannot answer all of my prayers.*
4   Realized that there were some things that even God could not change.*
5   Felt that even God has limits.*

### Religious and Spiritual Methods of Coping to Gain Control

***Collaborative religious coping***—*seeking control through a partnership with God in problem solving*

1   Tried to put my plans into action together with God.*
2   Worked together with God as a partner.*
3   Tried to make sense of the situation with God.*
4   Felt that God was working right along with me.*
5   Worked together with God to relieve my worries.*

***Active religious surrender***—*an active giving up of control to God in coping*

1   Did my best and then turned the situation over to God.*
2   Did what I could and put the rest in God's hands.*
3   Took control over what I could and gave the rest up to God.*
4   Tried to do the best I could and let God do the rest.*
5   Turned the situation over to God after doing all that I could.*

***Passive religious deferral***—*passive waiting for God to control the situation*

1   Didn't do much; just expected God to solve my problems for me.*
2   Didn't try much of anything; simply expected God to take control.*
3   Didn't try to cope; only expected God to take my worries away.*
4   Knew that I couldn't handle the situation; just expected God to take control.
5   Didn't try to do much; just assumed God would handle it.

***Pleading for direct intercession***—*seeking control indirectly by pleading to God for a miracle or divine intercession*

1   Pleaded with God to make things turn out okay.*
2   Prayed for a miracle.*
3   Bargained with God to make things better.*
4   Made a deal with God so that he would make things better.
5   Pleaded with God to make everything work out.

***Self-directing religious coping***—*seeking control directly through personal initiative rather than help from God*

1   Tried to deal with my feelings without God's help.*
2   Tried to make sense of the situation without relying on God.*
3   Made decisions about what to do without God's help.*
4   Depended on my own strength without support from God.
5   Tried to deal with the situation on my own without God's help.

## Religious and spiritual methods of coping to gain comfort and closeness to God

***Seeking spiritual support***—*searching for comfort and reassurance through God's love and care*

1   Sought God's love and care.*
2   Trusted that God would be by my side.*
3   Looked to God for strength, support, and guidance.*
4   Trusted that God was with me.
5   Sought comfort from God.

***Religious distraction***—*engaging in religious/spiritual activities to avoid focusing on the stressor*

1   Prayed to get my mind off of my problems.*
2   Thought about spiritual matters to stop thinking about my problems.*
3   Focused on religion to stop worrying about my problems.*
4   Went to church to stop thinking about this situation.
5   Tried to get my mind off my problems by focusing on God.

***Religious Purification***—*searching for spiritual cleansing through religious actions*

1   Confessed my sins.*
2   Asked forgiveness for my sins.*
3   Tried to be less sinful.*
4   Searched for forgiveness from God.
5   Asked for God to help me be less sinful.

***Spiritual Connection***—*experiencing a sense of connectedness with forces that transcend (rise above or go the limits of)*

1   Looked for a stronger connection with God.
2   Sought a stronger spiritual connection with other people.*
3   Thought about how my life is part of a larger spiritual force.*

4    Tried to build a strong relationship with a higher power.

5    Tried to experience a stronger feeling of spirituality.

**Spiritual discontent**—*expressing confusion and dissatisfaction with God's relationship to the person in the stressful situation*

1    Wondered whether God had abandoned me.*

2    Voiced anger that God didn't answer my prayers.*

3    Questioned God's love for me.*

4    Wondered if God really cares.

5    Felt angry that God was not there for me.

**Marking religious boundaries**—*clearly demarcating acceptable from unacceptable religious behavior and remaining within religious boundaries*

1    Avoided people who weren't of my faith.*

2    Stuck to the teachings and practices of my religion.*

3    Ignored advice that was inconsistent with my faith.*

4    Tried to stick with others of my own faith.

5    Asked clergy to remember me in their prayers.

**Religious and spiritual methods of coping to gain intimacy with others and closeness to God**

**Seeking support from clergy or congregation members**—*searching for comfort and reassurance through the love and care of congregation members and clergy*

1    Looked for spiritual support from clergy.*

2    Asked others to pray for me.*

3    Looked for love and concern from the members of my church.*

4    Sought support from members of my congregation.

5    Asked clergy to remember me in their prayers.

**Religious helping**—*attempting to provide spiritual support and comfort to others*

1    Prayed for the well-being of others.*

2    Offered spiritual support to family or friends.*

3    Tried to give spiritual strength to others.*

4    Tried to comfort others through prayer.

5    Tried to provide others with spiritual comfort.

*Interpersonal religious discontent—expressing confusion about and dissatisfaction with the relationship of clergy or congregation members to the person in the stressful situation*

1   Disagreed with what the church wanted me to do or believe.*
2   Felt dissatisfaction with the clergy.*
3   Wondered whether my church had abandoned me.*
4   Felt my church seemed to be rejecting or ignoring me.
5   Wondered whether my clergy were really there for me.

### Religious and spiritual methods of coping to achieve a life transformation

*Seeking religious direction—looking to religion for assistance in finding a new direction for living when the old one may no longer be viable*

1   Asked God to help me find a new purpose in life.*
2   Prayed to find a new reason to live.*
3   Prayed to discover my purpose in living.*
4   Sought new purpose in life from God.
5   Looked to God for a new direction in life.

*Religious conversion—looking to religion for a radical change in life*

1   Tried to find a completely new life through religion.*
2   Looked for a total spiritual reawakening.*
3   Prayed for a complete transformation of my life.*
4   Tried to change my whole way of life and follow a new path—God's path.
5   Hoped for a spiritual rebirth.

*Religious forgiving—looking to religion for help in shifting from anger, hurt, and fear to peace*

1   Sought help from God in letting go of my anger.*
2   Asked God to help me overcome my bitterness.*
3   Sought God's help in trying to forgive others.*
4   Asked God to help me be more forgiving.
5   Sought spiritual help to give up my resentments.

## Religious support

The religious support domain contains the following dimensions of social support:

- Emotional support received from fellow parishioners
- Emotional support given to others in one's congregation
- Negative interaction with coreligionists
- Anticipated support.

### *Religious support—long form*

*Emotional support received from others*

The following questions deal with the relationships you've had with the people in your congregation.

1  How often do the people in your congregation make you feel loved and cared for?

|   |   |   |   |
|---|---|---|---|
| 1 | Very often | 2 | Fairly often |
| 3 | Once in a while | 4 | Never |

2  How often do the people in your congregation listen to you talk about your private problems and concerns?

|   |   |   |   |
|---|---|---|---|
| 1 | Very often | 2 | Fairly often |
| 3 | Once in a while | 4 | Never |

3  How often do the people in your congregation express interest in and concern for your well-being?

|   |   |   |   |
|---|---|---|---|
| 1 | Very often | 2 | Fairly often |
| 3 | Once in a while | 4 | Never |

*Emotional support provided to others*

The following questions deal with things you may do for the people you worship with.

4  How often do you make the people in your congregation feel loved and cared for?

|   |   |   |   |
|---|---|---|---|
| 1 | Very often | 2 | Fairly often |
| 3 | Once in a while | 4 | Never |

5  How often do you listen to the people in your congregation talk about their private problems and concerns?

|   |   |   |   |
|---|---|---|---|
| 1 | Very often | 2 | Fairly often |
| 3 | Once in a while | 4 | Never |

6  How often do you express interest in and concern for the well-being of people you worship with?

1   Very often                     2   Fairly often
3   Once in a while                4   Never

*Negative interaction*

The contact we have with others is not always pleasant.

7  How often do the people in your congregation make too many demands on you?

1   Very often                     2   Fairly often
3   Once in a while                4   Never

8  How often are the people in your congregation critical of you and the things you do?

1   Very often                     2   Fairly often
3   Once in a while                4   Never

9  How often do the people in your congregation try to take advantage of you?

1   Very often                     2   Fairly often
3   Once in a while                4   Never

*Anticipated support*

These questions are designed to find out how much help the people in your congregation would be willing to provide if you need it in the future.

10  If you were ill, how much would the people in your congregation be willing to help out?

1   A great deal                   2   Some
3   A little                       4   None

11  If you had a problem or were faced with a difficult situation, how much comfort would the people in your congregation be willing to give you?

1   A great deal                   2   Some
3   A little                       4   None

12  If you needed to know where to go to get help with a problem you were having, how much would the people in your congregation be willing to help out?

1   A great deal                   2   Some
3   A little                       4   None

# References

Pargament, K., & Koenig, H. (1997). A comprehensive measure of religious coping: Development and initial validation of the RCOPE. Report presented at the Retirement Research Foundation, Chicago, IL.

Pargament, K., Smith, B., Koenig, H., & Perez, L. (1989). Patterns of positive and negative religious coping with major life stressors. *Journal for the Scientific Study of Religion, 37*(4), 711–725.

# Appendix I
## Spiritual Intelligence Assessment[1]

McMullen (2002) wrote that "if cognitive intelligence is about thinking and emotional intelligence is about feeling, then spiritual intelligence is about being" (p. 18). Zohar and Marshall (2002) proposed specific brain waves are consistent across the whole brain and associated with consciousness, and that consciousness connects cognitive events and perceptions into a meaningful whole (McMullen, 2002). The qualities of spiritual intelligence are wisdom and values such as courage, integrity, intuition, and compassion. According to McMullen (2002), "spirituality is an essential component of a holistic approach to life and work. It finds expression in creativity and all forms of the arts" (p. 18).

The Spiritual Intelligence Assessment can be given to anyone; it assesses possible spiritual experiences or practices. Respondents are instructed to circle the extent to which they experience or practice each item listed.

Respond to the following statements using:

| | | | | | |
|---|---|---|---|---|---|
| 1 | Many times a day | 2 | Every day | 3 | Most days |
| 4 | Some days | 5 | Once in a while | 6 | Almost never |

*To what extent can you say you experience the following:*

1   I feel a sense of awe and wonder at creation.

  1 2 3 4 5 6

2   I feel a sense of gratitude for life.

  1 2 3 4 5 6

3   I live in harmony with my deepest values and sense of meaning in life.

  1 2 3 4 5 6

4   I recognize the presence of the Divine in the world.

  1 2 3 4 5 6

5   I experience God's love for me, directly or through others.

  1 2 3 4 5 6

6   I experience a connection to the Source of All Life.

    1 2 3 4 5 6

7   I express and receive love and forgiveness in my relationships with others.

    1 2 3 4 5 6

8   I manage my emotions and behavior appropriately.

    1 2 3 4 5 6

9   I live with dignity and zeal.

    1 2 3 4 5 6

10  I have a spiritual community to whom I turn for support and help.

    1 2 3 4 5 6

11  I meditate or pray.

    1 2 3 4 5 6

12  I examine my thoughts, words, and actions and follow a program of self-improvement.

    1 2 3 4 5 6

13  I have regular dialogue with my spiritual coach, advisor, or rabbi.

    1 2 3 4 5 6

14  I have used my tradition as a source of strength, guidance, and direction.

    1 2 3 4 5 6

## Note

1 Reprinted from *Spiritual Intelligence Assessment* (p. xx), by Y. J. Kravitz, available at www.spiritualintelligence.com Copyright 2007 Rabbi Yaacov J. Kravitz, EdD, President and CEO, Center for Spiritual Intelligence, Melrose Park, CA.

## References

McMullen, B. (2002). Cognitive intelligence. *BMJ, 326*, 7376.

Zohar, D., & Marshall, I. (2002). *Spiritual intelligence: The ultimate intelligence*. New York: Bloomsbury.

# Index